Multiple Choice Questions in Clinical Pharmacology

MULTIPLE CHOICE QUESTIONS IN CLINICAL PHARMACOLOGY

Timothy GK Mant BSc, FFPM, FRCP
Medical Director,
Guy's Drug Research Unit, London, UK

Lionel D Lewis MA, MD, MRCP
Assistant Professor of Medicine and Pharmacology,
Dartmouth-Hitchcock Medical Center,
Lebanon, NH, USA

and

James M Ritter MA, DPhil, FRCP
Professor of Clinical Pharmacology,
United Medical and Dental Schools,
Guy's and St Thomas' Hospitals,
London, UK

A member of the Hodder Headline Group
LONDON • SYDNEY • AUCKLAND
Co-published in the USA by Oxford University Press, Inc., New York

First published in Great Britain by Edward Arnold 1995,
a member of the Hodder Headline PLC,
338 Euston Road, London NW1 3BH

Co-published in the United States of America by
Oxford University Press, Inc.,
198 Madison Avenue, New York, NY 10016
Oxford is a registered trademark of Oxford University Press

Whilst the advice and information in this book is believed to be true and
accurate at the date of going to press, neither the author nor the publisher
can accept any legal responsibility for any errors or omissions that may be
made. In particular (but without limiting the generality of the preceding
disclaimer) every effort has been made to check drug dosages; however, it
is still possible that errors have been missed. Furthermore, dosage
schedules are constantly being revised and new side effects recognised.
For these reasons the reader is strongly urged to consult the drug
companies' printed instructions before administering any of the drugs
recommended in this book.

British Library Cataloguing in Publication Data
A catalogue record for this book is available from the British Library

Library of Congress Cataloging-in-Publication Data
A catalog record for this book is available from the Library of Congress

ISBN 0 340 55932 2

5 6 7 8 9 10

Typeset in Helvetica and Adobe Garamond by
Anneset, Weston-super-Mare, Somerset
Printed and bound in Great Britain by
J W Arrowsmith Ltd, Bristol

CONTENTS

INTRODUCTION

Multiple choice questions are now ubiquitous in the final medical examinations. They provide a rapid method for testing a wide range of knowledge and marking is objective. The authors, all practicing physicians who have taught clinical pharmacology and therapeutics for many years, have based this book around the third edition of *Clinical Pharmacology and Therapeutics* not only to prepare students for their exams but also to emphasize those principles and facts which are the key to safe and effective prescribing.

The answers are related to the relevant section in *Clinical Pharmacology and Therapeutics (CPT)* . In addition there are brief annotations on each question.

Although this book can "stand alone", we hope students will read a section of the main textbook and then reinforce and revise their knowledge by self-testing themselves using the multiple choice questions (MCQ) book. At the end of the book is a practice examination of 60 questions. It covers the spectrum of topics that may be encountered in a final MB examination. We suggest that students use this as a "practice run" after finishing their revision of the subject as a whole. It is best to do it "blind" at one sitting lasting not more than 90 minutes. Many MCQ exams mark +2 for a correct response, 0 for no response and −1 for an incorrect response. Fifty per cent is the pass mark for the exam at the end of the book (i.e. 300/600 possible marks).

We thank the generations of UMDS students who have provided critical feedback, Dr Dipti Amin for her review of the questions and answers and Christine Hare for her word processing skills and patience.

1 GENERAL PRINCIPLES

1 The following drugs have been correctly paired with a measure of their pharmacodynamic effect:

(a) Warfarin – prolongation of prothrombin time
(b) Insulin – reduction in blood glucose
(c) Atenolol – reduction in exercise-induced tachycardia
(d) Morphine – pupil dilation
(e) Cimetidine – inhibition of gastric acid secretion

2 The following drugs exert their effects by combining with receptors and mimicking the effects of the natural mediator (i.e. are agonists):

(a) Tamoxifen
(b) Isoprenaline
(c) Morphine
(d) Terfenadine
(e) Captopril

3 The following drugs exert their principal effects by enzyme inhibition:

(a) Pyridostigmine
(b) Atropine
(c) Naloxone
(d) Digoxin
(e) Selegiline

4 The following drugs are reversible competitive antagonists:

(a) Suxamethonium
(b) Chlorpheniramine
(c) Ranitidine
(d) Phenoxybenzamine
(e) Naloxone

5 The following drugs are partial agonists:

(a) Isoprenaline
(b) Morphine
(c) Naloxone
(d) Buprenorphine
(e) Oxprenolol

6 The following drugs cause their effects via non-receptor (non-macro-molecular) mechanisms:

(a) Magnesium trisilicate
(b) Mannitol
(c) Ispaghula
(d) Dimercaprol
(e) Sumatriptan

1   **(a) True**   Pharmacodynamics is the study of the effects of drugs on
     (b) True   biological processes. One of the pharmacodynamic effects
     (c) True   of morphine is pupil constriction.
     (d) False
     (e) True

2   **(a) False** – Tamoxifen is an anti-oestrogen used in breast cancer
     (b) True – Isoprenaline is a β_1- and β_2-agonist
     (c) True – Morphine mimics the endogenous encephalins
     (d) False – Terfenadine is an antihistamine (H_1-blocker)
     (e) False – Captopril is an angiotensin-converting enzyme inhibitor

3   **(a) True** – Pyridostigmine is an inhibitor of acetylcholinesterase and is used
              in myasthenia gravis
     (b) False – Atropine blocks muscarinic receptors
     (c) False – Naloxone blocks opioid μ-receptors
     (d) True – Digoxin inhibits Na^+/K^+ adenosine triphosphatase (ATPase)
     (e) True – Selegiline is an MAO-B inhibitor used in Parkinson's disease

4   **(a) False** – Suxamethonium is an agonist that causes a seemingly para
              doxical inhibitory effect (neuromuscular blockade) by causing
              long-lasting depolarization of the neuromuscular junction
     (b) True – Chlorpheniramine is a histamine (H_1) antagonist
     (c) True – Ranitidine is a histamine (H_2) antagonist
     (d) False – Phenoxybenzamine is an irreversible α-receptor antagonist
     (e) True – Naloxone is a competitive antagonist at the morphine μ-receptor

5   **(a) False**   Partial agonists combine with receptors but are incapable of
     (b) False   eliciting a maximal reponse whatever their concentration.
     (c) False   Buprenorphine is a partial agonist at the morphine μ-receptor.
     (d) True   Oxprenolol is a partial agonist at the β-adrenoceptor.
     (e) True

6   **(a) True** – Magnesium trisilicate is an antacid which neutralizes gastric acid
     (b) True – Mannitol is an osmotic diuretic
     (c) True – Ispaghula is a bulk laxative
     (d) True – Dimercaprol is a chelating agent used in heavy metal poisoning
     (e) False – Sumatriptan is a $5HT_{1D}$ agonist used in migraine

7 The pharmacokinetic "half-life" of the following drugs resembles their pharmacodynamic "half-life":

(a) Salbutamol
(b) Phenelzine
(c) Dobutamine
(d) Omeprazole
(e) Cyclophosphamide

8 The clearance of a drug:

(a) Is the volume of plasma from which the drug is totally eliminated per unit time
(b) Is equal to the administration rate at steady state divided by the steady state plasma concentration
(c) Is a better measure of the efficiency of drug elimination than elimination half-life
(d) Does not include elimination by hepatic metabolism
(e) May be affected by renal function

9 For a drug that obeys first order (linear) kinetics and fits a one – compartment model of elimination:

(a) Its rate of elimination is proportional to its plasma concentration
(b) Following cessation of an intravenous infusion the plasma concentration declines exponentially
(c) The half-life is proportional to the dose
(d) The half-life is unaffected by renal function
(e) The composition of drug products excreted is independent of the dose

10 The apparent volume of distribution:

(a) Can be greater than the total body volume
(b) Is approximately 3 litres for most drugs in adults
(c) Is influenced by a drug's lipid solubility
(d) A large value indicates that a drug will be efficiently eliminated by hemodialysis
(e) Determines the peak plasma concentration after a bolus intravenous dose

11 The following drugs have an elimination half-life less than 4 hours in a healthy adult:

(a) Dopamine
(b) Heparin
(c) Amiodarone
(d) Gentamicin
(e) Diazepam

7 **(a) True**   The magnitude of pharmacological effect usually depends
   (b) False   directly on the concentration of drug (or active metabolites) in
   (c) True   the vicinity of their receptors. However, some drugs form
   (d) False   irreversible bonds at their sites of action so their effects
   (e) False   outlast their presence at these sites (e.g. alkylating agents).

8 **(a) True**   Clearance and not half life should be used as a measure of
   (b) True   the efficiency of drug elimination since $t_{\frac{1}{2}}$ is also dependent
   (c) True   on volume of distribution.
   (d) False
   (e) True

9 **(a) True**   Although the one compartment model is an oversimplification,
   (b) True   once absorption and distribution are complete many drugs
   (c) False   do obey first order elimination kinetics: See Fig. 1 below.
   (d) False
   (e) True

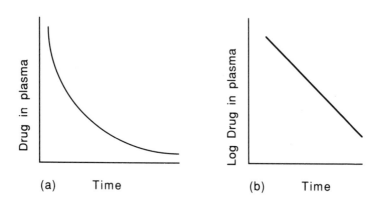

Fig. 1 One-compartment model. Plasma concentration–time curve following a bolus dose of drug plotted (a) arithmetically, or (b) semi-logarithmically. This drug fits a one-compartment model, i.e. its concentration falls exponentially with time

10 **(a) True**
   (b) False   Volume of distribution dose/C_0. C_0 is the plasma concentration
   (c) True   at time zero calculated by extrapolation following a bolus
   (d) False   intravenous injection.
   (e) True

11 **(a) True** – Dopamine, 2 minutes
   (b) True – Heparin, 0.5–2.5 hours
   (c) False – Amiodarone, 28–45 days
   (d) True – Gentamicin, 2 hours
   (e) False – Diazepam, 20–50 hours

12 In repeated (multiple) dosing:
- (a) If the dosing interval is much greater than the half-life little if any accumulation occurs
- (b) It takes approximately five half-lives to reach 50% of the steady state concentration
- (c) If a drug is administered once every half-life the peak plasma concentration will be double the trough concentration
- (d) The use of a bolus loading dose reduces the time taken to reach steady state
- (e) In renal impairment the dosing interval should be increased when prescribing gentamicin

13 The following drugs obey non-linear (dose-dependent) elimination pharmacokinetics in therapeutic doses:
- (a) Salicylate
- (b) Heparin
- (c) Phenytoin
- (d) Ethanol
- (e) Cefuroxime

14 The following undergo enterohepatic cycling:
- (a) Estrogens
- (b) Cefuroxime
- (c) Rifampicin
- (d) Gentamicin
- (e) Ciprofloxacin

15 The oral bioavailability of a drug:
- (a) Is a measure of the extent to which it enters the systemic circulation
- (b) May be influenced by changing the excipient from calcium sulphate to lactose
- (c) Is determined by comparing the area under the plasma concentration time curve (AUC) following oral and intravenous administration
- (d) May be reduced by hepatic enzyme induction
- (e) Two preparations of a drug may have similar bioavailability but have different peak concentrations

16 The following are examples of prodrugs:
- (a) Levodopa
- (b) Azathioprine
- (c) Benorylate
- (d) Sulfasalazine
- (e) Frusemide

12 **(a) True**   It takes approximately three half-lives to approximate steady
     (b) False   state (87.5% of steady state). After four half-lives it is 93%
     (c) True   and after five half-lives 96.9%.
     (d) True
     (e) True

13 **(a) True**   Implications of non-linear kinetics include: the time taken to
     (b) True   eliminate 50% of a dose increases with increasing dose and
     (c) True   the concept of half-life is meaningless; once the drug elimina-
     (d) True   tion process is saturated, a relatively modest increase in dose
     (e) False   dramatically increases the amount of drug in the body.

14 **(a) True**   Enterohepatic cycling is when a drug is excreted into the bile,
     (b) False   reabsorbed from the intestine and returned via the portal sys-
     (c) True   tem to the liver to be recycled.
     (d) False
     (e) False

15 **(a) True**   See *CPT*, Chapter 4, pp. 30–32. Although the bioavailability of
     (b) True   two preparations may be the same, the kinetics can be very
     (c) True   different as seen in some immediate and slow release
     (d) True   formulations.
     (e) True

16 **(a) True**   – Levodopa $\rightarrow$ dopamine
     (b) True   – Azathioprine $\rightarrow$ 6-mercaptopurine
     (c) True   – Benorylate $\rightarrow$ paracetamol + aspirin
     (d) True   – Sulfasalazine $\rightarrow$ aminosalicylate + sulfapyridine
     (e) False

17 The following oral drugs do not require absorption from the gut to exert a therapeutic effect:
   (a) Acarbose
   (b) Methionine
   (c) Cholestyramine
   (d) Sulfasalazine
   (e) Vancomycin

18 Drug absorption following oral administration:
   (a) Is most commonly through passive diffusion
   (b) Occurs predominantly in the colon
   (c) Is usually complete within 60 minutes
   (d) Non-polar lipid-soluble drugs are absorbed more readily than polar water-soluble drugs
   (e) Peptides are well absorbed following oral administration

19 The following drugs are absorbed predominantly through active transport systems:
   (a) Paracetamol
   (b) Phenytoin
   (c) Levodopa
   (d) Methyldopa
   (e) Lithium

20 The systemic bioavailability of the following oral drugs is increased if taken in the fasting state:
   (a) Oxytetracycline
   (b) Ampicillin
   (c) Levodopa
   (d) Acetylsalicylic acid/salicylates
   (e) Griseofulvin

21 The following drugs are usefully administered by the sublingual route:
   (a) Digoxin
   (b) Carbamazepine
   (c) Captopril
   (d) Buprenorphine
   (e) Glyceryl trinitrate

22 The following drugs are usefully administered by the rectal route for their systemic effect:
   (a) Indomethacin
   (b) Sulfasalazine
   (c) Metronidazole
   (d) Glycerin
   (e) Diazepam

17   **(a) True** – Acarbose is a competitive inhibitor of intestinal α-glucosidases

         (b) False – Methionine, an antidote to paracematol poisoning, acts not in the gastrointestinal tract but predominantly in the liver where it repletes glutathione which inactivates the toxic paracetamol metabolite

         (c) True – Cholestyramine is a bile acid binding resin which indirectly lowers plasma low density lipoprotein (LDL) cholesterol hence it has a systemic effect without systemic drug absorption

         (d) True – Sulfasalazine delivers 5-aminosalicylate to the colon where it has a local action in inflammatory bowel disease

         (e) True – Vancomycin kills toxin producing *Clostridium difficile*, the cause of pseudomembranous colitis within the bowel

18   **(a) True**   Most oral drugs are absorbed by passive diffusion in the small

         (b) False   bowel. In general low molecular weight, high lipid solubility

         (c) False   and lack of charge encourage absorption. Most peptides are

         (d) True   broken down enzymically.

         (e) False

19   **(a) False**   Active transport requires specific carrier-mediated energy con-

         (b) False   suming mechanisms. Naturally occurring polar nutrients and

         (c) True   aliments including sugars, amino-acids and vitamins are

         (d) True   absorbed by active or facilitated transport mechanisms. Drugs

         (e) True   that are analogs of such molecules compete for uptake. Further examples include methotrexate and 5-fluorouracil.

20   **(a) True**   Food and drink dilute the drug and can adsorb or otherwise

         (b) True   compete with it. Transient increases in hepatic blood flow

         (c) False   such as occur after a meal may result in greater availability of

         (d) False   drug by reducing pre-systemic hepatic metabolism.

         (e) False

21   **(a) False**   Sublingual administration is an effective means of causing

         (b) False   systemic effects, and has distinct advantages over oral

         (c) False   administration (i.e. the drug is swallowed) for drugs with

         (d) True   pronounced presystemic metabolism, providing direct and

         (e) True   rapid access to the systemic circulation bypassing intestine and liver. See *CPT*, Chapter 4, p. 34.

22   **(a) True** – Rectal indomethacin administered at night is useful in reducing early morning stiffness in rheumatoid arthritis

         (b) False – Rectal sulfasalazine is used for its local effect in inflammatory bowel disease

         (c) True – Rectal metronidazole is well absorbed (and much less expensive than the intravenous preparation)

         (d) False – Glycerin suppositories exert a local effect to stimulate defecation

         (e) True – Rectal diazepam is used to control convulsions when venous access is difficult (as may be the case in children)

23 The following drugs are applied to the skin to produce systemic effect:
  (a) Glyceryl trinitrate
  (b) Estradiol
  (c) Lignocaine
  (d) Hydrocortisone
  (e) Nicotine

24 Intramuscular injection:
  (a) Rate of absorption is enhanced by exercise
  (b) Rate of absorption is greater from the deltoid injection site than the gluteus maximus site
  (c) If administered to the buttock should be in the upper outer quadrant
  (d) Should usually be no greater than 0.5 ml
  (e) Is an appropriate route of administration for the decanoate ester of fluphenazine

25 The following drugs are commonly associated with phlebitis when given via the intravenous route:
  (a) Erythromycin
  (b) Hydrocortisone
  (c) Diazepam
  (d) 50% glucose
  (e) 5% glucose

26 The following are metabolized in hepatic smooth endoplasmic reticulum:
  (a) Levodopa
  (b) Tyramine
  (c) Theophylline
  (d) Suxamethonium
  (e) 6-mercaptopurine

27 The following are substrates for cytochrome P_{450}:
  (a) Procainamide
  (b) Erythromycin
  (c) Phenobarbitone
  (d) Adrenaline
  (e) Warfarin

28 The following drugs are acetylated:
  (a) Dapsone
  (b) Debrisoquine
  (c) Gentamicin
  (d) Isoniazid
  (e) Hydralazine

23 **(a) True** – Transdermal GTN is used in ischemic heart disease and is being investigated in premature labor
    (b) True – Transdermal estradiol is used for hormone replacement therapy in menopausal women
    (c) False – Local lignocaine is used for its local anesthetic action (e.g. for intravenous cannulation in children)
    (d) False – Topical hydrocortisone is used for a local anti-inflammatory action without the disadvantage of systemic corticosteroids
    (e) True – Nicotine is used to assist cigarette smokers to abstain

24 **(a) True** – Exercise and local massage increase the rate of absorption
    (b) True – Transport from the injection site is governed by muscle blood flow – deltoid > vastus lateralis > gluteus maximus
    (c) True – This avoids the risk of sciatic nerve palsy
    (d) False – Up to 5 ml is acceptable in the buttock
    (e) True – This depot preparation is slowly hydrolyzed in muscle to release active drug and is used to improve compliance in schizophrenic patients

25 **(a) True**
    (b) False
    (c) True – An oily emlusion, (diazemuls ™) reduces this complication
    (d) True
    (e) False

26 **(a) False** – Levodopa is decarboxylated to dopamine in central neurones
    (b) False – Tyramine is metabolized by monoamine oxidase (MAO) in intestine, liver, kidney and nervous tissue. MAO is a mitochondrial enzyme
    (c) True
    (d) False – Suxamethonium is metabolized by plasma cholinesterase
    (e) False – Purines (e.g. 6-mercaptopurine) are metabolized by xanthine oxidase which is a non-microsomal enzyme

27 **(a) False** – Procainamide is acetylated
    (b) True – Erythromycin as well as being metabolized by cytochrome P_{450} enzymes inhibits the metabolism of other drugs subject to cytochrome P_{450} metabolism (e.g. warfarin, theophylline and terfenadine)
    (c) True – Phenobarbitone also induces cytochrome P_{450} enzymes
    (d) False – Adrenaline is a catecholamine and is metabolized by catechol-O-methyltransferase which is present in the cytosol
    (e) True – Warfarin has a narrow therapeutic index

28 **(a) True**
    (b) False – Debrisoquine is a "marker" drug for hydroxylator status and is metabolized by cytochrome P_{450} enzymes
    (c) False – Gentamicin is eliminated unchanged by the kidney
    (d) True
    (e) True

29 The following cause hepatic enzyme induction:

(a) Rifampicin
(b) Carbamazepine
(c) Ethanol
(d) Phenobarbitone
(e) Penicillin

30 The following inhibit cytochrome P_{450}:

(a) Cimetidine
(b) Erythromycin
(c) Digoxin
(d) Ketoconazole
(e) Ciprofloxacin

31 The following are subject to extensive presystemic metabolism:

(a) Chlorpheniramine
(b) Phenytoin
(c) Ciprofloxacin
(d) Morphine
(e) Verapamil

32 The following decrease the rate of gastric emptying

(a) Myocardial infarction
(b) Migraine
(c) Myxedema
(d) Duodenal ulcer
(e) Metoclopramide

33 Cardiac failure:

(a) Reduces the bioavailability of thiazide diuretics
(b) Increases the volume of distribution of lignocaine
(c) Has little effect on the volume of distribution of frusemide
(d) Decreases the terminal half-life of lignocaine
(e) Decreases the terminal half-life of gentamicin

29 **(a) True** – Rifampicin is a broad spectrum antibiotic used in tuberculosis and Legionnaire's disease
   (b) True – Carbamazepine is an anticonvulsant
   (c) True
   (d) True – Phenobarbitone is an anticonvulsant
   (e) False – Penicillin is predominantly eliminated unchanged in the urine

   Drug interactions secondary to hepatic enzyme induction and inhibition are clinically significant when there is a close correlation between plasma concentration and effect, and a steep dose response curve

30 **(a) True** – Cimetidine is an H_2 blocker which blocks gastric acid secretion
   (b) True – Erythromycin is a macrolide antibacterial drug
   (c) False – Digoxin is predominantly eliminated unchanged in the urine
   (d) True – Ketoconazole is an antifungal agent
   (e) True – Ciprofloxacin is a fluoroquinolone antibacterial drug

31 **(a) False**   Presystemic metabolism occurs in the gastrointestinal mucosa
   (b) False   and liver; presystemic (first pass) metabolism necessitates
   (c) False   high oral doses in comparison with the intravenous dose.
   (d) True   Such drugs usually exhibit marked interindividual variability
   (e) True   in effective dose.

32 **(a) True** – Pain decreases the rate of gastric emptying
   (b) True
   (c) True
   (d) False
   (e) False – Metoclopramide accelerates gastric emptying

33 **(a) True** – The absorption of thiazides is reduced by 30–40%
   (b) False – The volume of distribution of lignocaine is reduced probably because of decreased tissue perfusion
   (c) True – The distribution volume of frusemide is largely confined to the vascular compartment
   (d) False – Is prolonged predominantly due to decreased hepatic perfusion
   (e) False – Glomerular filtration is reduced in cardiac failure and hence the elimination half-life of gentamicin is prolonged (i.e. not decreased)

34 In severe renal failure:
   (a) Gastric pH decreases
   (b) The "therapeutic range" for phenytoin decreases
   (c) Drug distribution to the brain is decreased
   (d) Smaller maintenance doses of digoxin are required
   (e) Inulin clearance gives a more accurate estimate of glomerular filtration rate than creatinine clearance

35 The following statements are correct:
   (a) The kidneys receive approximately 20% of the cardiac output
   (b) In healthy young adults approximately 130 ml/min of protein-free filtrate is formed at the glomeruli
   (c) Non-protein bound drug of molecular weight < 66 000 passes into the filtrate
   (d) Potentially saturable mechanisms for active secretion of both acids and bases exist in the proximal tubule
   (e) Low lipid solubility favors tubular reabsorption

36 The following are actively secreted into the tubular fluid in the proximal segment:
   (a) Inulin
   (b) Probenecid
   (c) Penicillin
   (d) Para-aminohippuric acid (PAH)
   (e) Cimetidine

37 The following drugs must be avoided in severe renal failure (glomerular filtration rate < 10 ml/min):
   (a) Prednisolone
   (b) Amoxycillin
   (c) Bumetanide
   (d) Metformin
   (e) Oxytetracycline

38 The following can impair renal function:
   (a) Naproxen
   (b) Ranitidine
   (c) Iodine-containing contrast media
   (d) Captopril
   (e) Amphotericin B

34   **(a) False** – Gastric pH increases

     (b) True – The ratio of unbound : bound phenytoin rises in renal failure. It is unbound drug which is active and the laboratory assay for phenytoin measures whole blood concentration (bound and unbound)

     (c) False – The blood–brain barrier becomes functionally less of a barrier to drug distribution in severe renal failure. This may be the reason for the increased incidence of confusion associated with cimetidine in renal failure

     (d) True – The volume of distribution is decreased and renal clearance reduced

     (e) True – Inulin clearance is the "gold standard" measure of glomerular filtration rate

35   **(a) True**   The kidney is involved to some degree in the elimination of

     (b) True   virtually every drug or drug metabolite in man. High lipid

     (c) True   solubility and the unionized state favor reabsorption.

     (d) True

     (e) False

36   **(a) False**   Unlike glomerular filtration, tubular secretion can eliminate

     (b) True   drugs efficently even if they are protein bound. Competition

     (c) True   can occur (e.g. probenecid and penicillin).

     (d) True

     (e) True

37   **(a) False**

     (b) False – Reduce dose; rashes more common

     (c) False – May need very high doses for any effect

     (d) True – Increased risk of lactic acidosis

     (e) True – Direct nephrotoxicity, anti-anabolic, increases blood urea

38   **(a) True** – Non steroidal anti-inflammatory drugs (NSAIDs) cause salt and water retention, and reduce renal blood flow by inhibition of prostacyclin and prostaglandin E_2 synthesis in patients with renal compromise. This disrupts autoregulation of renal blood flow and GFR thus preventing the normal physiological mechanism which ensures preferential perfusion of the functioning kidney. NSAIDs are less commonly associated with papillary necrosis or interstitial nephritis

     (b) False

     (c) True – Radiographic contrast media cause a transient decrease in GFR. The mechanism is unknown

     (d) True – Angiotensin-converting enzyme (ACE) inhibitors, although often effective in treating heart failure and hypertension in patients with renal disease, can impair renal function. They must be avoided in bilateral renal artery stenosis

     (e) True – Can cause acute tubular necrosis and renal tubular acidosis

39 The following drugs should be avoided in hepatic failure:
   (a) Spironolactone
   (b) Chlorpromazine
   (c) Lactulose
   (d) Aluminum hydroxide
   (e) Metronidazole

40 Monitoring drug concentrations of the following drugs is recognized as a valuable supplement to clinical monitoring:
   (a) Cyclophosphamide
   (b) Warfarin
   (c) Gentamicin
   (d) Lithium
   (e) Cyclosporin

41 The following are associated with a decreased clearance of theophylline:
   (a) Cirrhosis
   (b) Heart failure
   (c) Gilbert's syndrome
   (d) Concurrent phenobarbitone
   (e) Smoking

42 In pregnancy:
   (a) Most drugs cross the placenta by active transport
   (b) Ionized drugs cross the placenta more easily than unionized drugs
   (c) Drugs that reduce placental blood flow can reduce birth weight
   (d) The fetal blood–brain barrier is not developed until the second half of pregnancy
   (e) The human placenta metabolizes endogenous steroids

43 The following drugs are confirmed teratogens in humans:
   (a) Alcohol
   (b) Warfarin
   (c) Isotretinoin
   (d) Paracetamol
   (e) Amoxycillin

39   **(a) False**   – Spironolactone, an aldosterone antagonist, is effective in reducing ascites. Secondary hyperaldosteronism is a feature of hepatic failure

     (b) True   – Chlorpromazine is hepatotoxic and can precipitate coma

     (c) False   – Lactulose is commonly used to reduce ammonia production

     (d) True   – Aluminum hydroxide causes constipation which indirectly increases plasma ammonia

     (e) False

40   **(a) False**

     (b) False   – Warfarin therapy is monitored by measurement of prothrombin time (INR)

     (c) True   – Gentamicin "peak" concentrations (30 minutes after dose) correlate with efficacy, trough concentrations correlate with toxicity. Aminoglycosides are associated with irreversible ototoxicity and reversible nephrotoxicity

     (d) True   – Insidious increases in serum lithium concentrations can lead to coma and convulsions

     (e) True   – Not only does cyclosporin show marked interindividual variability but also compliance is a particular problem in children. Deterioration in renal function post transplant may reflect either graft rejection possibly associated with low cyclosporin concentrations or toxicity from excessive concentrations

41   **(a) True**   Theophylline has a narrow therapeutic window and plasma

     (b) True   concentrations are affected by many factors. High concentra-

     (c) False   tions are associated with convulsions and arrhythmias. Of

     (d) False   major concern is the asthmatic on oral theophylline who may

     (e) False   take additional theophylline because of deteriorating asthma who is then given intravenous theophylline in casualty. Phenobarbitone induces P_{450} and increases theophylline clearance; so does smoking.

42   **(a) False**   Most drugs cross the placenta (a cellular membrane) by

     (b) False   passive diffusion down a concentration gradient. Lipid

     (c) True   solubility enhances transport across membranes and drugs in

     (d) True   the unionized state are more lipid soluble. The human

     (e) True   placenta possesses multiple enzymes.

43   **(a) True**   – The risk of having an abnormal baby is about 10% in mothers drinking 30–60 ml ethanol per day rising to 40% in chronic alcoholics

     (b) True   – Warfarin has been associated with nasal hypoplasia and chondrodysplasia when given in the first trimester and with CNS abnormalites and haemorrhagic complications in later pregnancy. Neonatal haemorrhage is difficult to prevent because of the immature enzymes in fetal liver and low stores of vitamin K

     (c) True   – Isotretinoin is a teratogen. Effective contraception must be used for at least 1 month before, during, and at least 1 month after oral treatment

     (d) False   – The minor analgesic of choice in pregnancy

     (e) False   – Commonly used to treat urinary tract infection in pregnancy

44 During pregnancy:

    (a) Gastric emptying and small intestinal motility are reduced
    (b) Blood volume increases
    (c) Plasma volume increases
    (d) Predominantly water-soluble drugs will have a larger apparent volume of distribution
    (e) Phenytoin metabolism is inhibited

45 During pregnancy:

    (a) Renal plasma flow increases
    (b) Glomerular filtration rate increases
    (c) Digoxin excretion increases
    (d) Lithium excretion increases
    (e) Gentamicin excretion increases

46 The following are believed safe in pregnancy:

    (a) Penicillins
    (b) Cephalosporins
    (c) Fluoroquinolones
    (d) Aminoglycosides
    (e) Erythromycin

47 The following are appropriate in the management of dyspepsia in the second and third trimester:

    (a) Low roughage diet
    (b) Avoidance of fresh fruit and vegetables
    (c) Small, frequent meals
    (d) Misoprostol
    (e) Alginates

48 The following drugs do not cross the placenta in significant amounts:

    (a) Heparin
    (b) Warfarin
    (c) Corticosteroids
    (d) Sodium valproate
    (e) Pethidine

49 The use of phenytoin in pregnancy:

    (a) Is absolutely contraindicated
    (b) Is associated with cleft lip and palate
    (c) The therapeutic blood concentration of total drug is lower than in the non-pregnant state
    (d) Is associated with ataxia if an excessive dose is used
    (e) Requires oral vitamin D supplements

44   **(a) True**   – This is of little consequence unless rapid drug action is required.
                     Vomiting associated with pregnancy occasionally makes oral
                     administration impractical
     (b) True   – Blood volume in pregnancy increases by one-third
     (c) True   – Plasma volume increases from 2.5 to 4 litres at term and is
                     disproportionate to the expansion in red cell mass so the
                     hematocrit falls
     (d) True   – Edema, which at least one third of women experience during
                     pregnancy, may add up to 8 litres to the volume of extracellular
                     water. For water-soluble drugs (which usually have a relatively
                     small volume of distribution) this increases the volume of
                     distribution
     (e) False – Metabolism of drugs by the pregnant liver is increased

45   **(a) True**   Excretion of drugs via the kidney increases because renal
     (b) True   plasma flow almost doubles and the glomerular filtration rate
     (c) True   increases by two-thirds during pregnancy.
     (d) True
     (e) True

46   **(a) True**
     (b) True
     (c) False – Minimal experience, animal data discouraging
     (d) False – The fetal VIIIth nerve is more sensitive to aminoglycoside toxicity
     (e) True

47   **(a) False**   Non-drug treatment – reassurance, small frequent meals and
     (b) False   advice on posture should be pursued in the first instance.
     (c) True   Misoprostol, which is an analog of prostaglandin E_1 causes
     (d) False   abortion.
     (e) True

48   **(a) True**   – Accumulating evidence suggests this is also true for the low
                     molecular weight heparins (which may become anticoagulants of
                     choice in pregnancy)
     (b) False
     (c) False
     (d) False
     (e) False

49   **(a) False**   Epilepsy in pregnancy can lead to fetal and maternal
     (b) True   morbidity/mortality through convulsions. Although all anti-
     (c) True   convulsants are teratogenic the risk of untreated epilepsy is
     (d) True   much greater to the mother and fetus than drug-induced
     (e) False   teratogenicity.

50 The following drugs are appropriate for managing hypertension diagnosed in pregnancy:

    (a) Bendrofluazide
    (b) Atenolol
    (c) Labetalol
    (d) ACE inhibitors
    (e) Methyldopa

51 The following are absolutely contraindicated in pregnancy:

    (a) Salbutamol
    (b) Corticosteroids
    (c) General anesthesia
    (d) Quinine
    (e) Sucralfate

52 In neonates relative to adults:

    (a) Gastric acid is reduced
    (b) Fat content (as a percentage of body weight) is low
    (c) Plasma albumin concentration is low
    (d) The blood–brain barrier is more permeable
    (e) The glomerular filtration rate is reduced

53 The following drugs should be avoided during breast feeding:

    (a) Amiodarone
    (b) Carbamazepine
    (c) Ciprofloxacin
    (d) Cytotoxics
    (e) Ranitidine

54 The following drugs suppress lactation:

    (a) Anthraquinones (e.g. senna)
    (b) Bromocriptine
    (c) Frusemide
    (d) Salbutamol
    (e) Metronidazole

50 **(a) False**   See *CPT*, Chapter 9, p. 80 and Chapter 25, pp. 302–303.
    (b) True
    (c) True
    (d) False
    (e) True

51 **(a) False** – Commonly used to treat asthma and occasionally premature labor
    (b) False – Minimal problems when given by inhalation or in short courses (e.g. to help mature fetal lung) and although cleft palate and congenital cataract have been attibuted to large systemic doses of corticosteroids the benefit of treatment usually outweighs the risk
    (c) False – Although there is an increased risk of spontaneous abortion associated with general anesthesia a causal link is uproven and in most circumstances failure to operate would have dramatically increased the risk to mother and fetus
    (d) False – Falciparum malaria has a high mortality in pregnancy
    (e) False – Sucralfate is not absorbed

52 **(a) True**   Neonates are not miniature adults in terms of drug handling
    (b) True   because of differences in body constitution, drug absorption,
    (c) True   distribution, metabolism, excretion and sensitivity to adverse
    (d) True   reactions.
    (e) True

53 **(a) True** – Significant concentration in breast milk and there is a theoretical risk from iodine release
    (b) False – Minimal concentration in breast milk
    (c) True – High concentration in breast milk, animal experiments suggest damage to growing joints
    (d) True – Avoid breast feeding
    (e) False

54 **(a) False** – But may cause diarrhea in infant
    (b) True
    (c) True
    (d) False
    (e) False – But gives milk an unpleasant taste

55 The following properties of a drug encourage their presence in breast milk:

   (a) High lipid solubility
   (b) Unionized state
   (c) Low molecular weight
   (d) Weak base
   (e) Short half-life

56 The following are appropriate in the management of acute severe asthma in a 5-year-old child:

   (a) Nebulized β_2-agonists
   (b) Systemic corticosteroids
   (c) Rectal diazepam
   (d) Systemic ipratropium
   (e) Systemic chlorpheniramine

57 A "normal" man of 75 in comparison with a "normal" adult of 35:

   (a) Is more likely to be on regular drug therapy
   (b) Is more prone to sedation with benzodiazepines
   (c) Has a higher endogenous production of creatinine
   (d) Has an increased liability to allergic reactions
   (e) Usually requires a lower dose of warfarin to achieve anticoagulation

58 The following drugs may precipitate acute retention of urine in the elderly:

   (a) Gliclazide
   (b) Frusemide
   (c) Thioridazine
   (d) Amitriptyline
   (e) Ampicillin

55　(a) **True**　　The total dose of drug in breast milk ingested by the infant is
　　(b) **True**　　usually too small to cause problems (with some notable
　　(c) **True**　　exceptions, see Table 1). The infant should be monitored
　　(d) **True**　　clinically if β-adrenoceptor antagonists are prescribed to the
　　(e) **False**　　mother. Milk is midly acid, so weak bases accumulate in it.

Table 1　Some drugs to be avoided during breast feeding.

Vitamin A/Retinoid analogs	Cyclosporin
Amiodarone	Cytotoxics
Stimulant laxatives	Ergotamine
Benzodiazepines	Octreotide
Chloramphenicol	Sulfonylureas
Ciprofloxacin	Thiazide diuretics
Combined oral contraceptives	

56　(a) **True**
　　(b) **True**　 – A 5-day course of systemic corticosteroids is often sufficent
　　(c) **False** – Potentially fatal
　　(d) **False**
　　(e) **False** – Potentially fatal

57　(a) **True**
　　(b) **True**
　　(c) **False** – One reason why plasma creatinine is a less reliable indicator of
　　　　　　　　　　renal function in the elderly is that endogenous creatinie
　　　　　　　　　　production is reduced.
　　(d) **True**
　　(e) **True**

58　(a) **False** – Gliclazide, a short-acting sulfonylurea, is commonly prescribed to
　　　　　　　　　　elderly diabetics who are inadequately controlled by diet alone
　　(b) **True**
　　(c) **True**　 – Thioridazine, a phenothiazine which is commonly used to treat
　　　　　　　　　　restlessness and agitated depression in the elderly, has
　　　　　　　　　　anticholinergic effects which may lead to retention of urine
　　(d) **True**　 – Amitryptyline, a sedative tricyclic antidepressent, also has
　　　　　　　　　　anticholinergic effects.
　　(e) **False**

59 The half-life of the following drugs is increased in the elderly:
  (a) Gentamicin
  (b) Glibenclamide
  (c) Lithium
  (d) Dextropropoxyphene
  (e) Diazepam

60 The following drugs should not be used in those over 75 years old:
  (a) Captopril
  (b) Chlorpropamide
  (c) Streptokinase
  (d) Doxycycline
  (e) Fluoxetine

61 A woman of 75 is more likely to have the following adverse effects than a woman of 25:
  (a) Confusion during treatment with cimetidine
  (b) Dystonia during treatment with metoclopramide
  (c) Gastrointestinal hemorrhage during treatment with indomethacin
  (d) Increased incidence of postural hypotension during phenothiazine therapy
  (e) Increased risk of agranulocytosis during clozapine therapy

62 The following are "type A" adverse reactions (i.e. a consequence of the drug's normal pharmacological effect):
  (a) Atenolol and fatigue
  (b) Chlorpromazine and hepatotoxicity
  (c) Naproxen and gastrointestinal hemorrhage
  (d) Cyclophosphamide and neutropenia
  (e) Diazepam and sedation

63 Stopping treatment with the following drugs may lead to adverse effects due to drug withdrawal:
  (a) Prednisolone
  (b) Clonidine
  (c) Lorazepam
  (d) Metoprolol
  (e) Ergotamine

64 The following adverse reactions are associated with the drugs named:
  (a) Oral contraception – gastrointestinal hemorrhage
  (b) Heparin – thrombocytopenia
  (c) Cimetidine – gynecomastia
  (d) Thiazide diuretics – impotence
  (e) Prednisolone – osteomalacia

59 **(a) True**   – Related to the decrease in GFR associated with aging
    (b) True   – Related to the decrease in GFR associated with aging
    (c) True   – Related to the decrease in GFR associated with aging
    (d) True   – Related to the decrease in GFR associated with aging
    (e) True   – Due to the increase in volume of distribution and probably also reduced metabolism

60 **(a) False**
    (b) True   – Chlorpropamide may cause prolonged hypoglycemia
    (c) False
    (d) False   – Doxycycline is a unique tetracycline in that it is not affected by renal function
    (e) False   Has fewer anticholinergic effects than most antidepressants

61 **(a) True**
    (b) False   – Most common in young women
    (c) True
    (d) True   – Impairment of cardiovascular reflexes to erect posture in the elderly is exaggerated by phenothiazines
    (e) True

62 **(a) True**   See *CPT*, Chapter 11, p. 94–95.
    (b) False
    (c) True
    (d) True
    (e) True

63 **(a) True**   – Prolonged corticosteroid therapy leads to adrenal atrophy and insufficiency. Risks are minimized by the use of steroid cards, using systemic corticosteroids for the minimum period necessary and gradual withdrawal after prolonged therapy. Atrophy may persist for years after stopping corticosteroid therapy and may only be revealed during "stress" (e.g. acute illness/surgery)
    (b) True   – Rebound hypertension
    (c) True   – Benzodiazepines causes psychological and physical addiction
    (d) True
    (e) False

64 **(a) False**   – Oral contraceptive use is associated wth thromboembolism
    (b) True
    (c) True
    (d) True
    (e) False   – Corticosteroid therapy is associated with osteoporosis. Prolonged use of some anticonvulsants (e.g. phenytoin) is associated with osteomalacia

65 The following are examples of type I hypersensitivity reaction:
  (a) Penicillin-induced anaphylactic shock
  (b) Methyldopa-induced Coombs' postive hemolytic anemia
  (c) Hydralazine-induced systemic lupus erythematosus
  (d) Amiodarone-induced photosenstivity skin rashes
  (e) Terfenadine- induced ventricular tachycardia

66 The following drugs are associated with erythema multiforme:
  (a) Phenytoin
  (b) Cyclophosphamide
  (c) Salbutamol
  (d) Halothane
  (e) Co-trimoxazole

67 The following drugs are recognized as causing aplastic anemia:
  (a) Chloramphenicol
  (b) Atenolol
  (c) Loperamide
  (d) Clozapine
  (e) Mianserin

68 The following combinations outside the body (e.g. in infusion bag) cause drug
    inactivation
  (a) Penicillin and hydrocortisone
  (b) Phenytoin and 5% glucose
  (c) Sodium bicarbonate and calcium chloride
  (d) Erythromycin and 0.9% normal saline
  (e) Heparin and 5% glucose

69 Individuals who are "slow acetylators" (ie: have relatively low activities of
    hepatic N-acetyltransferase):
  (a) Have prevalence of 5–10% amongst Causasians in the the UK
  (b) Are more likely to develop aplastic anemia whilst being treated with
       clozapine
  (c) Are more likely to develop hepatotoxicity after a paracetamol overdose
  (d) Are more likely to develop a lupus-like syndrome during hydralazine
       therapy
  (e) Are more likely to develop peripheral neuropathy during isoniazid therapy

70 The following drugs can produce hemolysis in patients with glucose
    6-phosphate dehydrogenase (G6PD) deficiency:
  (a) Dapsone
  (b) Paracetamol
  (c) Primaquine
  (d) Co-trimoxazole
  (e) Ciprofloxacin

65 (a) **True**
    (b) **False** – A type II reaction
    (c) **False** – A type III reaction
    (d) **False** – A type IV reaction
    (e) **False** – Related to high terfenadine blood concentrations, often as a
        result of drug interaction

66 (a) **True** – Also associated with acne, coarse facies, hirsutism and toxic
        epidermal necrolysis
    (b) **False**
    (c) **False**
    (d) **False**
    (e) **True** – Usually due to the sulfamethoxazole but may also be caused by
        trimethoprim

67 (a) **True**   See *CPT*, Chapter 11, p. 103.
    (b) **False**
    (c) **False**
    (d) **True**
    (e) **True**

68 (a) **True** – Inactivation of penicillin
    (b) **True** – Precipitates
    (c) **True** – Precipitates
    (d) **False**
    (e) **False**

69 (a) **False**   Approximately 45% of Caucasians are slow acetylators.
    (b) **False**   Examples of drugs acetylated include: isoniazid, hydralazine
    (c) **False**   phenelzine, dapsone and procainamide. The usual "marker" is
    (d) **True**   the dapsone metabolite ratio in the plasma. The isoniazid
    (e) **True**   peripheral neuropathy can be prevented by prophylactic use
                      of pyridoxine.

70 (a) **True**   The gene for G6PD is located on the X chromosome. G6PD
    (b) **False**   deficiency is more common in people from Mediterranean
    (c) **True**   countries.
    (d) **True**
    (e) **True**

71 Drug-induced exacerbations of acute porphyria:
   (a) Are usually precipitated by enzyme inhibitors (e.g. cimetidine)
   (b) Are often precipitated by a single dose of drug
   (c) Are accompanied by increased urinary excretion of 5-aminolevulinic acid (ALA) and porphobilinogen
   (d) May be precipitated by ethanol
   (e) May be precipitated by rifampicin

72 Abnormal pseudocholinesterase:
   (a) Is typically inherited as a Mendelian dominant
   (b) Results in malignant hyperthermia following exposure to suxamethonium
   (c) Causes warfarin resistance
   (d) Leads to prolonged paralysis following suxamethonium
   (e) Is associated with Alzheimer's disease

73 Phase I studies (i.e. initial studies of drugs in man):
   (a) Usually require authorization by the Committee on Safety Medicines
   (b) The control group is usually the current drug of choice for the proposed indication
   (c) Always use the oral route of administration
   (d) Only commence after all animal studies have been completed
   (e) Are usually performed in terminal patients

74 The Committee on Safety of Medicines (CSM):
   (a) Is an independent group of clinicians, clinical pharmacologists, toxicologists, pathologists and others who advise the drug licensing authority
   (b) Is financed directly by the UK pharmaceutical industry
   (c) Considers the quality, safety and efficacy of medicinal products
   (d) considers the investigation, monitoring and response to adverse reactions once a drug has been licenced
   (e) Appoints the local committees on ethical practice

75 The following adverse reactions should be reported to the CSM using the yellow prepaid letter card:
   (a) A transient mild skin rash in a patient taking a new non-steriodal anti-inflammatory drug marked with a "▼" in the *British National Formulary*
   (b) Aggravation of asthma in a known asthmatic with the drug of question "a"
   (c) A convulsion following pertussis vaccination
   (d) Acute anaphylactic shock following intravenous penicillin
   (e) Aplastic anemia associated with clozapine

71 **(a) False**   The acute porphyrias are due to hereditary abnormalities in
    (b) True   heme biosynthesis and may be precipitated by many drugs
    (c) True   (see list in *British National Formulary*), expecially inducers of
    (d) True P_{450} enzymes.
    (e) True

72 **(a) False**   The usual response to a single intravenous dose of
    (b) False   suxamethonium is muscular paralysis for about six minutes.
    (c) False   The effect is brief due to hydrolysis of suxamethonium by
    (d) True   plasma pseudocholinesterase. Approximately 1 in 2500
    (e) False   patients have abnormal pseudocholinesterase which may
                       result in prolonged paralysis for 2 hours. Inheritance is
                       Mendelian recessive.

73 **(a) False** – Only requires approval of the MCA (Medicine Control Agency) if
                     patients are the volunteers
    (b) False – Placebo is the usual control
    (c) False
    (d) False
    (e) False – Phase I studies are usually performed in healthy male adults
                     aged 18–35 years

74 **(a) True**   The CSM in practice is the regulatory review board of the UK
    (b) False   who advise when certificates to perform clinical trials should
    (c) True   be issued to pharmaceutical companies and advising,
    (d) True   following review of all the data from a submission, on the
    (e) False   granting of a product license which will allow the company to
                       market the drug.

75 **(a) True**   See *CPT*, Chapter 11. pp. 96–97.
    (b) True
    (c) True
    (d) True
    (e) True

2 NERVOUS SYSTEM

76 The following are causes of insomnia:

    (a) Day-time exercise
    (b) Left ventricular failure
    (c) Caffeine
    (d) Depression
    (e) Fluoxetine

77 Benzodiazepines:

    (a) Are the hypnotics of choice in most patients
    (b) Should only be used as hypnotics for a maximum of 2–4 weeks
    (c) Suppress REM sleep
    (d) Act by binding to the GABA receptor–chloride channel complex and facilitate the opening of the channel in the presence of GABA
    (e) Are anxiolytic

78 Benzodiazepine dependence and withdrawal syndrome:

    (a) Is caused by large doses taken for prolonged periods
    (b) Fits can occur in the first week after withdrawal
    (c) The full withdrawal picture usually appears after an interval of 3–8 weeks
    (d) Perceptual distortions are characteristic
    (e) Shorter acting benzodiazepines are less likely to cause dependence and should be substituted for long-acting benzodiazepines when withdrawing a patient from benzodiazepines

79 Diazepam:

    (a) Has a half-life of less than 20 hours
    (b) Can cause anterograde amnesia
    (c) Is effective in terminating acute dystonia caused by metoclopramide
    (d) Never causes fatal overdose
    (e) The major site of metabolism is the liver

80 Temazepam:

    (a) Has a shorter half-life than diazepam
    (b) Potentiates the effects of alcohol
    (c) Causes no "hangover" effect 10 hours post-dosing
    (d) Is not addicitive
    (e) In more potent than lorazepam

81 Chlormethiazole:

    (a) Is not absorbed orally
    (b) Has a half-life of approximately 15 minutes
    (c) In cirrhosis the bioavailability is increased about 10-fold
    (d) High doses cause cardiovascular and respiratory depression
    (e) Is antagonized by ethanol

76 **(a) False**   It is important to exclude causes of insomnia that require
    (b) True   treatment (e.g. pain, dyspnea, frequency of micturition,
    (c) True   caffeine and depression). Some individuals need little
    (d) True   sleep, shortened sleep time is common in the elderly.
    (e) True

77 **(a) True**   Benzodiazepines, whilst being much safer than the
    (b) True   barbiturates, still have the problems of dependence, potentia-
    (c) True   tion of alcohol, respiratory depression in overdose and
    (d) True   suppressing REM sleep.
    (e) True

78 **(a) True**
    (b) True
    (c) False – The full withdrawal picture usually appears after an interval of
              3–8 days
    (d) True
    (e) False – It is common practice to substitute shorter-acting with longer-
              acting benzodiazepines (e.g. temazepam → diazepam) to assist
              withdrawal

79 **(a) False** – Up to 50 hours, the active desmethyl metabolite has a half-life of
              36–200 hours
    (b) True
    (c) True
    (d) False – Usually in combination with alcohol or other drugs
    (e) True

80 **(a) True** – 5–6 hours in comparison with 20–50 hours
    (b) True – This combination is a common cause of fatal overdose as well
              as disinhibited behavior which may lead to crime or road traffic
              accidents
    (c) False – Patients must be warned not to drive or operate heavy machin-
              ery if affected
    (d) False
    (e) False

81 **(a) False**
    (b) False
    (c) True – This results from decreased first pass metabolism
    (d) True – Fatalities have occurred because of poorly supervised intra-
              venous infusions. Constant rate infusions lead to accumulation
    (e) False

82 Promethazine:
- (a) Is a GABA agonist
- (b) Is available without prescription
- (c) Causes dry mouth, constipation and reduced sweating
- (d) Liver failure is an absolute contraindication
- (e) May cause hallucinations

83 Zopiclone:
- (a) Is an ultra short-acting benzodiazepine
- (b) Is the hypnotic of choice in a breast-feeding mother
- (c) Is a more effective anticonvulsant than clonazepam
- (d) Is associated with drug dependence
- (e) Can cause confusion

84 The following drugs may mimic some of the common clinical features of schizophrenia:
- (a) Levodopa
- (b) Salbutamol
- (c) LSD
- (d) Diamorphine
- (e) Methylenedioxymethylamphetamine (MDMA, ecstasy)

85 Blockade of central D_2-receptors:
- (a) Parallels the clinical efficacy of most antipsychotic drugs
- (b) Induces extra-pyramidal effects
- (c) Repeated administration of D_2-antagonists causes an increase in D_2-agonist sensitivity due to an increase in abundance of these receptors
- (d) Repeated administration of D_2- antagonists may lead to tardive dyskinesia
- (e) Causes a decrease in cardiac output

86 The general principles of management of schizophrenia include:
- (a) Treatment should be started in hospital promptly after diagnosis
- (b) Chlorpromazine is frequently successful on its own in acute psychotic episodes
- (c) Concomitant anticholinergics should be routinely prescribed
- (d) Once first-rank symptoms have been relieved most patients can return home on low dose antipsychotic maintenance treatment
- (e) Risperidone is an effective alternative to chlorpromazine

87 Chlorpromazine:
- (a) Has an antidopaminergic action on the extra-pyramidal system
- (b) Has an antidopaminergic action on the mesolimbic system
- (c) Has an antidopaminergic action on the chemoreceptor trigger zone
- (d) Has moderate antimuscarinic properties
- (e) Has α-adrenoreceptor blocking properties

82 **(a) False** – Promethazine is an H1-antihistamine
    (b) True
    (c) True – Anticholingergic effects
    (d) True – May cause coma
    (e) True

83 **(a) False**   Zopiclone is a non-benzodiazepine hypnotic which enhances
    (b) False   GABA activity.
    (c) False
    (d) True
    (e) True

84 **(a) True**   Occasionally drug-induced hallucinations/psychosis may be
    (b) False   mistaken for schizophrenia. The hypothesis that chronic
    (c) True   cannabis use and LSD can precipitate schizophrenia is
    (d) False   unproven.
    (e) True

85 **(a) True**   Prolonged use of D2-receptor blockers is associated with the
    (b) True   onset of tardive dyskinesia which may involve structural brain
    (c) True   damage and is often irreversible.
    (d) True
    (e) False

86 **(a) True**
    (b) True
    (c) False
    (d) True
    (e) True – Risperidone is a recently introduced anti-psychotic agent which
            appears to be more effective against negative symptoms than
            chlorpromazine.

87 **(a) True** – Leading to extra-pyramidal side effects
    (b) True – This may be the site of antipsychotic action
    (c) True – Leading to anti-emetic effect
    (d) True
    (e) True

88 Indications for phenothiazines such as chlorpromazine include:
   (a) Mania
   (b) Emesis
   (c) Severe agitation and panic
   (d) Aggressive and violent behavior
   (e) Malignant neuroleptic syndrome

89 Adverse effects associated with phenothiazines include:
   (a) Dry mouth
   (b) Blurred vision
   (c) Postural hypotension
   (d) Impaired temperature control
   (e) Jaundice

90 Contraindications to phenothiazines include:
   (a) Huntington's disease
   (b) Concomitant morphine
   (c) Asthma
   (d) Hepatic impairment
   (e) Bone marrow depression

91 Chlorpromazine:
   (a) Has an oral bioavailability of over 90%
   (b) Has a low volume of distribution (approx. 100 ml/kg)
   (c) Is predominantly eliminated via the kidneys as unchanged chlorpromazine
   (d) Of the chlorpromazine in plasma, 90–95% is bound to plasma proteins
   (e) Usually once daily administration is adequate

92 Butyrophenones (e.g. haloperidol) in comparison to phenothiazines (e.g. chlorpromazine) are generally:
   (a) Less sedating
   (b) Less hypotensive
   (c) Less antimuscarinic
   (d) Have more extra-pyramidal effects
   (e) Not contraindicated in epilepsy

93 Flupenthixol:
   (a) Is particularly effective in mania
   (b) May be given once every 2–4 weeks via the intramuscular route for chronic schizophrenia
   (c) Is less sedating than chlorpromazine
   (d) Is more prone than chlorpromazine to produce extra- pyramidal toxicity
   (e) Should not be used in patients with porphyria

88   **(a) True**
     (b) True
     (c) True
     (d) True
     (e) False – Anti-psychotic drugs may cause maligant neuroleptic syndrome. This rare syndrome (hyperthermia, varying conscious level, rigidity and autonomic dysfunction) may be treated with dantrolene or bromocriptine

89   **(a) True** – Anticholinergic
     (b) True – Anticholinergic
     (c) True – Peripheral α-adrenoceptor blockade
     (d) True – Hypothermia in cold weather, hyperthermia in hot weather
     (e) True – Jaundice occurs in 2–5% of patients taking chlorpromazine. It is due to intrahepatic cholestasis and is a hypersenstivity phenomenon associated with eosinophilia

90   **(a) False** – Often used to reduce movement and mental disorders in Huntington's disease
     (b) False
     (c) False
     (d) True
     (e) True – May cause blood dyscrasias which can be fatal

91   **(a) False** – Oral bioavailabilty is about 30%
     (b) False – Volume of distribution is large, approximately 22 l/kg
     (c) False – Metabolism predominately by hepatic microsomes. Over 70 metabolites have been identified
     (d) True
     (e) True

92   **(a) True**   Haloperidol is sometimes preferred to phenothiazines for rapid
     (b) True   control of hyperactive psychotic states. It may be conveniently
     (c) True   given in this indication by the intramuscular route.
     (d) True
     (e) False

93   **(a) False**   Depot intramuscular preparations such as flupenthixol
     (b) True   decanoate are valuable in the management of schizophrenia
     (c) True   for maintenance therapy to ensure compliance which is often
     (d) True   poor in such patients.
     (e) True

94 Clozapine:
   (a) Has weak D_2-blocking activity
   (b) Is effective in up to 60% of patients who have not responded to phenothiazines
   (c) Is effective against negative as well as positive symptoms
   (d) Rarely causes tardive dyskinesia
   (e) Causes blood dyscrasias more commonly than other antipsychotics

95 The following drugs raise synaptic and/or total brain monoamines:
   (a) Reserpine
   (b) Amitriptyline
   (c) Imipramine
   (d) Phenelzine
   (e) Amphetamine

96 Tricyclic antidepressants:
   (a) Are more effective in endogenous rather than reactive depression
   (b) Are particularly effective when the depression is associated with psychomotor and physiological changes
   (c) Onset of therapeutic action is approximately 2 weeks after starting therapy
   (d) Are effective in the management of panic disorder
   (e) Are used for the treatment of nocturnal enuresis in children

97 Antidepressants with sedative properties include:
   (a) Amitriptyline
   (b) Clomipramine
   (c) Dothiepin
   (d) Protriptyline
   (e) Mianserin

98 The following are consistent with tricyclic antidepressant overdose:
   (a) Dilated pupils
   (b) Hyperreflexia
   (c) Sinus tachycardia
   (d) Widened QRS on the ECG
   (e) Convulsions

99 The following effects are associated with tricyclic antidepressants:
   (a) Hypersalivation
   (b) Constipation
   (c) Aggravation of narrow angle glaucoma
   (d) Dry skin due to loss of sweating
   (e) Fine tremor

94 **(a) True**   Neutropenia or agranulocytosis develops in up to 3% of
   (b) True   patients taking clozapine for 1 year. Although dystonias and
   (c) True   tardive dyskinesias are rare, clozapine is associated with fits
   (d) True   in 3–4% of patients and rarely cardiovascular collapse.
   (e) True

95 **(a) False**   Reserpine depletes neuronal stores of noradrenaline (NA)
   (b) True   and 5-hydroxytryptamine (5HT) and causes depression.
   (c) True   Tricyclic drugs of the amitriptyline type raise synaptic stores of
   (d) True   NA and 5HT and are antidepressant. Monoamine oxidase
   (e) True   inhibitors which increase total brain NA and 5HT are also
                    antidepressant. Amphetamine and cocaine raise synaptic NA
                    and alter mood but are not antidepressant.

96 **(a) True**   See *CPT*, Chapter 17.
   (b) True
   (c) True
   (d) True
   (e) True

97 **(a) True**   The less sedative tricyclic and related antidepressants include
   (b) True   desipramine, imipramine, lofepramine and nortriptyline.
   (c) True   Protriptyline is a stimulant. The more sedative drugs are
   (d) False   preferred for agitated and anxious patients, whilst the less
   (e) True   sedative are preferred in withdrawn patients.

98 **(a) True**   Tricyclic antidepressant overdoses are commonly fatal.
   (b) True   Patients may die from cardiac arryhthmias, convulsions or
   (c) True   direct CNS depression leading to respiratory arrest/asphyxia.
   (d) True   See *CPT*, Chapter 50.
   (e) True

99 **(a) False** – Anticholinergic action leads to dry mouth
   (b) True – Anticholinergic action
   (c) True – Anticholinergic action
   (d) True – Anticholinergic action
   (e) True – Sympathomimetic action

100 The following are contraindications to imipramine therapy:

    (a) Asthma
    (b) Epilepsy
    (c) Recent myocardial infarction
    (d) Unpaced heart block
    (e) Porphyria

101 Amitriptyline:

    (a) Is highly lipid soluble
    (b) Is highly protein bound
    (c) Has a low volume of distribution (approx. 100 ml/kg body weight)
    (d) Blocks uptake of monoamines into cerebral and other neurones
    (e) Delays gastric emptying

102 Mianserin:

    (a) Inhibits MAO
    (b) Is a powerful anticholinergic agent
    (c) Is less sedative than imipramine
    (d) Causes orthostatic hypotension
    (e) During therapy the blood count should be monitored

103 Fluoxetine:

    (a) Selectively blocks neuronal uptake of noradrenaline
    (b) Is more cardiotoxic than imipramine
    (c) Is less sedative than amitriptyline
    (d) Is associated with nausea and dyspepsia
    (e) Has a short elimination half-life of 1–2 hours

104 Phenelzine:

    (a) Is a reversible selective inhibitor of MAO-B
    (b) Onset of therapeutic effect is usually within 1 week
    (c) Is ineffective if used alone in the treatment of depression
    (d) Is sometimes effective in reducing hypochondriacal and hysterical symptoms
    (e) Is more likely to cause a hypertensive crisis when an indirectly acting sympathomimetic (e.g. ephedrine) is given concurrently than a directly acting sympathomimetic (e.g. adrenaline)

105 Moclobemide:

    (a) Is a reversible selective inhibitor of MAO-A
    (b) is effective adjunct therapy in Parkinson's disease
    (c) Has a longer duration of MAO inhibition compared to phenelzine after stopping therapy
    (d) Causes dry mouth in over 50% of patients
    (e) Is less likely than phenelzine to cause a food (tyramine) interaction

100 **(a) False**   See *CPT*, Chapter 17, p. 172.
      (b) True
      (c) True
      (d) True
      (e) True

101 **(a) True**   Amitriptyline is a sedative tricyclic antidepressant which is
      (b) True   usually administered as a single nocte dose.
      (c) False
      (d) True
      (e) True

102 **(a) False**   Mianserin is a sedative antidepressant which has little anti-
      (b) False   cholinergic and cardiac toxicity (which may help reduce death
      (c) False   from overdose) but is associated with orthostatic hypotension
      (d) True   and blood dyscrasias.
      (e) True

103 **(a) False**   Fluoxetine is a selective serotonin (5HT) re-uptake inhibitor. It
      (b) False   is safer in overdose and causes fewer antimuscarinic side
      (c) True   effects than the tricyclic antidepressants.
      (d) True
      (e) False

104 **(a) False**   Phenelzine (and isocarboxazid and tranylcypromine) are
      (b) False   irreversible non-selective MAO inhibitors.
      (c) False
      (d) True
      (e) True   – Adrenaline is metabolized by catechol-*O*-methyltransferase

105 **(a) True**
      (b) False   – Selegiline, a MAO-B inhibitor, is used in Parkinson's disease
      (c) False
      (d) False   – No anticholinergic action (cf. tricyclic antidepressants)
      (e) True   – Reversible, competitive, selective MAO inhibitor

106 The following foodstuffs/chemicals can cause a hypertensive/hyperthermic reaction during non-selective monamine oxidase inhibitor therapy:

(a) Cheese
(b) Yoghurt
(c) Beer
(d) Marmite™
(e) Grouse

107 Lithium toxicity can be precipitated by:

(a) Sodium depletion
(b) Thiazide therapy
(c) ACE inhibitors
(d) Non-steroidal anti-inflammatory drugs
(e) Atenolol

108 Therapeutic drug monitoring of plasma concentrations of the following drugs is routinely indicated:

(a) Amitriptyline
(b) Phenelzine
(c) Lofepramine
(d) Lithium
(e) Tryptophan

109 Tricyclic antidepressant therapy should not be started within 14 days of therapy with:

(a) Phenelzine
(b) Isocarboxazid
(c) Tranylcypromine
(d) Moclobemide
(e) Carbamazepine

110 Parkinsonism is associated with the following drugs/poisons:

(a) Paraquat
(b) Quinine
(c) Phenothiazines
(d) Ethanol
(e) Carbon monoxide

111 Muscarinic antagonists (e.g. benzhexol, benztropine):

(a) Are predominantly used in Parkinsonism caused by antipsychotic drugs
(b) Are least effective in the treatment of tremor
(c) Are ineffective in the management of postencephalitic Parkinsonism
(d) Must not be used with levodopa
(e) May cause confusion in the elderly

106 **(a) True**   Patients on MAO inhibitors should be given a treatment card
    (b) True   which lists necessary precautions. Interactions with foodstuffs,
    (c) True   many proprietary preparations and prescribed drugs may
    (d) True   cause a hypertensive crisis. Phenotolamine and/or labetalol
    (e) True   are effective treatment for such a reaction.

107 **(a) True**   Lithium salts have a narrow therapeutic index. Lithium concen-
    (b) True   trations may rise insidiously and once adverse effects such as
    (c) True   tremor, ataxia, dysarthria and nystagmus develop treatment
    (d) True   must be stopped whilst the serum lithium (avoid lithium
    (e) False   heparin tubes to collect plasma) is measured urgently.

108 **(a) False**   See *CPT*, Chapter 8.
    (b) False
    (c) False
    (d) True
    (e) False – Tryptophan has been withdrawn from general use because of its
            association with eosinophilic myalgic syndrome

109 **(a) True**   – Irreversible non-selective MAO inhibitor
    (b) True   – Irreversible non-selective MAO inhibitor
    (c) True   – Irreversible non-selective MAO inhibitor
    (d) False – Reversible selective MAO inhibitor
    (e) False – An anticonvulsant, not an MAO inhibitor

110 **(a) False**   The toxic causes of Parkinsonism include phenothiazines,
    (b) False   butyrophenones, manganese, carbon monoxide poisoning and
    (c) True   MPTP, an illicit "designer drug". Although alcohol withdrawal
    (d) False   causes a tremor, alcohol and β-blockers reduce benign
    (e) True   essential tremor.

111 **(a) True**   Muscarinic antagonists are effective in the treatment of
    (b) False   Parkinsonian tremor and to a lesser extent rigidity. They have
    (c) False   minimal effects on bradykinesia. Although more commonly
    (d) False   prescribed to counteract antipsychotic-drug induced
    (e) True   Parkinsonism they may be used alone in idiopathic
                 Parkinsonism and posten cephalitic Parkinsonism if tremor
                 is the predominant symptom.

112 The following enhance central dopaminergic activity:

    (a) Inhibition of MAO-B
    (b) Bromocriptine
    (c) Apomorphine
    (d) Haloperidol
    (e) Intravenous dopamine

113 Levodopa:

    (a) Can enter nerve terminals
    (b) Is oxidized by MAO to form dopamine
    (c) Is antagonized by bromocriptine
    (d) Antagonizes the hypotensive effects of β-blockers
    (e) May cause dystonic reactions

114 Levodopa:

    (a) Is the amino acid precurser of dopamine
    (b) Improves bradykinesia and rigidity more than tremor
    (c) Levodopa therapy should be initiated with a loading dose
    (d) Levodopa should be taken on an empty stomach
    (e) Involuntary movements and psychiatric complications are common unwanted effects

115 Bromocriptine:

    (a) Stimulates release of endogenous dopamine
    (b) Stimulates postsynaptic D_2 receptors
    (c) Is used in conjunction with levodopa–dopa decarboxylase inhibitors
    (d) Has an antiemetic action
    (e) Is drug of first choice in newly diagnosed idiopathic Parkinsonism

116 Selegiline:

    (a) Selectively inhibits MAO-B
    (b) The most common adverse effect is postural hypotension
    (c) Is principally eliminated unchanged in the urine
    (d) Cannot be prescribed concurrently with levodopa
    (e) Cannot be prescribed concurrently with amantadine

117 The following drugs reduce spasticity in patients with upper motor neurone lesions:

    (a) Imipramine
    (b) Metoclopramide
    (c) Diazepam
    (d) Baclofen
    (e) Dantrolene

112 **(a) True**   Parkinsonism arises because of deficient dopaminergic trans-
    (b) True   mission. Acetylcholine is antagonistic to dopamine within the
    (c) True   striatum.
    (d) False
    (e) False

113 **(a) True**   Levodopa (unlike dopamine) can enter nerve terminals in the
    (b) False   basal ganglia where it undergoes decarboxylation to form
    (c) False   dopamine.
    (d) False
    (e) True

114 **(a) True**   The dose of levodopa is titrated upwards balancing efficacy
    (b) True   against adverse effects. Nausea and vomiting are reduced by
    (c) False   the addition of a dopa decarboxylase inhibitor and taking the
    (d) False   drug after food.
    (e) True

115 **(a) False**   Bromocriptine is used as an adjunct with levodopadopa
    (b) True   decarboxylase combinations in patients with severe
    (c) True   motor fluctuations. There is great individual variation
    (d) False   in its efficacy. Currently it is used in late stages of
    (e) False   Parkinsonism (clinical trials in early disease are ongoing).

116 **(a) True**   Selegeline, an MAO-B inhibitor may slow disease progression
    (b) False   in idiopathic Parkinson's disease. It usually allows dose
    (c) False   reduction and prolongs the duration of action of levodopa.
    (d) False   Oral selegeline is well absorbed (100%) and extensively
    (e) False   metabolized in the liver. Rarely hypertension has been
                       reported. Amantidine (which stimulates release of endogenous
                       dopamine) potentiates its anti-Parkinson effects.

117 **(a) False**   Treatment of spasticity is seldom very effective, but physio-
    (b) False   therapy or limited surgical release procedures have some
    (c) True   place. The drugs used to reduce spasticity have considerable
    (d) True   limitations. Diazepam is sedative, baclofen is less sedative at
    (e) True   equieffective doses but can cause vertigo, nausea and
                       hypotension. Intrathecal baclofen is currently being evaluated.
                       Dantrolene is less useful for spasticity as it markedly reduces
                       muscle power. It is used in the management of neuroleptic
                       malignant syndrome and malignant hyperthermia.

118 Tardive dyskinesia:

    (a) Occurs in about 15% of patients treated with neuroleptic drugs for over 2 years

    (b) Stopping treatment results in slow improvement in approximately 40% of patients

    (c) Dyskinesia may initially worsen after discontinuing treatment

    (d) Consists of rapid involuntary movements of the limbs

    (e) Is treated with botulinum toxin A

119 In myasthenia gravis:

    (a) Therapy is usually initiated with neostigmine

    (b) Thymectomy may be beneficial

    (c) Corticosteroids and azathioprine reduce circulating T cells

    (d) There is increased sensitivity to suxamethonium

    (e) Corticosteroids can worsen or improve weakness

120 Severe weakness in a patient with myasthenia gravis may be potentiated by:

    (a) Spontaneous deterioration in the natural history of the disease

    (b) Excessive anticholinesterase drug

    (c) Acute infection

    (d) Aminoglycosides

    (e) Amitriptyline

121 Ethosuximide:

    (a) Is effective in petit mal absences

    (b) Sedation is the most common adverse effect

    (c) Concurrent phenytoin therapy is contraindicated

    (d) Plasma concentration monitoring is routinely required

    (e) Has a shorter half-life in children than adults

122 Phenytoin is indicated in:

    (a) Febrile convulsions

    (b) Petit mal absences

    (c) Tonic clonic (grand mal) seizures

    (d) Partial (focal) seizures

    (e) Psychomotor attack

123 The following are recognized adverse effects associated with phenytoin therapy:

    (a) Ataxia

    (b) Dysarthria

    (c) Acne

    (d) Hyperkalemia

    (e) Macrocytic anemia

118 (a) **True**   Tardive dyskinesia is thought to result from the development
    (b) **True**   of "denervation hypersensitivity" in dopaminergic postsynaptic
    (c) **True**   receptors of the nigrostriatal pathway following chronic recep-
    (d) **False**   tor blockade by neuroleptics. It is therefore due to a relative
    (e) **False**   preponderance of dopaminergic effects. Botulinum toxin A is
                      one of the neurotoxins produced by *Clostridium botulinum* and
                      is used to treat blepharospasm and certain other dystonias. It
                      blocks the release of acetylcholine at the neuromuscular
                      junction and is given by local intramuscular injection. This is a
                      specialist field!

119 (a) **True**   Myasthenia gravis is a syndrome of increased muscle
    (b) **True**   fatiguability and weakness of striated muscle and results from
    (c) **True**   an autoimmune process with antibodies to nicotinic
    (d) **False**   acetylcholine receptors.
    (e) **True**

120 (a) **True**   Clinically the distinction between a deficiency (myasthenic
    (b) **True**   crisis) or an excess (cholinergic crisis) may be difficult and
    (c) **True**   improvement with an injection of the very short-acting anti-
    (d) **True**   cholinesterase edrophonium is diagnostic of myasthenic crisis.
    (e) **False**   Because of its short duration of action, any deterioration of a
                      cholinergic crisis is unlikely to have serious consequences
                      although facilities for artificial ventilation must be available.
                      NB: cholinesterase inhibitors cause pupillary constriction.

121 (a) **True**   Ethosuximide is effective in petit mal absences. It is usually
    (b) **False**   continued into adolescence and then gradually withdrawn.
    (c) **False**   Side-effects are rare but dizziness, nausea and epigastric
    (d) **False**   discomfort are occasionally troublesome.
    (e) **True**

122 (a) **False**   Phenytoin is one of the drugs of choice in the treatment of
    (b) **False**   tonic clonic (grand mal) and partial (focal) seizures, including
    (c) **True**   psychomotor attack.
    (d) **True**
    (e) **True**

123 (a) **True**   High blood concentrations of phenytoin produce a cerebellar
    (b) **True**   syndrome, involuntary movements and sedation. Macrocytic
    (c) **True**   anemia which responds to folate is common. Rashes, fever,
    (d) **False**   hepatitis, gum hypertrophy, hirsutism and lymphadenopathy
    (e) **True**   lare all well recognized adverse effects of phenytoin.

124 The pharmacokinetics of phenytoin are characterized by:

    (a) Wide interindividual variation
    (b) Less than 10% systemic bioavailability if taken by mouth with food
    (c) Two populations – fast and slow acetylators
    (d) The half-life is not affected by dose
    (e) Once daily dosing is adequate

125 The ratio of unbound to bound phenytoin is increased by:

    (a) Uremia
    (b) Pregnancy
    (c) Concurrent sodium valproate therapy
    (d) Concurrent heparin therapy
    (e) Migraine

126 Carbamazepine:

    (a) Inhibits GABA transaminase
    (b) inhibits its own metabolism
    (c) Is effective in temporal lobe epilepsy
    (d) Inhibits the metabolism of warfarin
    (e) Once daily dosing is adequate

127 The following adverse effects are associated with carbamazepine therapy:

    (a) Trigeminal neuralgia
    (b) Sedation
    (c) Dizziness
    (d) Diplopia
    (e) Hyponatremia

128 Clonazepam:

    (a) Is a glutamate receptor antagonist
    (b) Is indicated in motor seizures of childhood
    (c) Is indicated in status epilepticus
    (d) Is ineffective when given by mouth
    (e) Has a half-life of approximately 30 minutes

129 Sodium valproate:

    (a) Is a dopamine antagonist
    (b) Is indicated in tonic–clonic epilepsy
    (c) The commonest adverse effects are dizziness and sedation
    (d) Rarely causes hepatic necrosis
    (e) Is safe in pregnancy

130 Vigabatrin:

    (a) Is a structural analog of GABA
    (b) Increases the brain concentration of GABA
    (c) Is first line treatment in tonic–clonic epilepsy
    (d) May cause hallucinations and paranoia
    (e) Is excreted unchanged by the kidney

124 (a) True
    (b) False
    (c) False
    (d) False
    (e) True

Age, body weight, sex and in particular, saturable metabolism which is under polygenic control, contribute to the wide variation in handling of phenytoin.

125 (a) True
    (b) True
    (c) True
    (d) False
    (e) False

Unbound, free drug is active. The plasma concentration of phenytoin includes both bound and unbound drug. If this ratio is altered, the therapeutic range should be adjusted accordingly.

126 (a) False
    (b) False
    (c) True
    (d) False
    (e) False

In addition to its effectiveness in all forms of epilepsy except absence seizures, carbamazepine is effective in trigeminal neuralgia. It induces its own metabolism hence the half-life after a single dose is 25–60 hours but on chronic dosing this falls to 10 hours.

127 (a) False
    (b) True
    (c) True
    (d) True
    (e) True

Carbamazepine commonly causes adverse effects but these are seldom severe. They are particularly troublesome early in treatment and may resolve without alteration of dose which is probably related to the induction of its own metabolism. Hyponatremia is caused by stimulation of antidiuretic hormone secretion.

128 (a) False
    (b) True
    (c) True
    (d) False
    (e) False

Benzodiazepines are anticonvulsant but are often sedative at effective doses and on prolonged use tolerance to their anti-epileptic properties tends to develop. Clonazepam is used intravenously in the treatment of status epilepticus and orally as maintenance therapy in a wide variety of seizure types, in particular, the motor seizures of childhood including absences and infantile spasms. It has a half-life of 30 hours.

129 (a) False
    (b) True
    (c) False
    (d) True
    (e) False

Sodium valproate is effective against several forms of epilepsy. Adverse effects most commonly involve the alimentary system. These include nausea, vomiting and abdominal pain (which may be reduced by enteric coated tablets). Use in pregnancy is associated with increased neural tube defects.

130 (a) True
    (b) True
    (c) False
    (d) True
    (e) True

Vigabatrin is reserved for the treatment of epilepsy unsatisfactorily controlled by more established drugs.

131 The following anticonvulsants induce the metabolism of estrogen and can lead to unwanted pregnancies in women using oral contraception:
   (a) Carbamazepine
   (b) Phenytoin
   (c) Sodium valproate
   (d) Phenobarbitone
   (e) Primidone

132 An 18-year-old man is admitted to casualty in status epilepticus. There is a history of three previous unexplained blackouts in the last year. The following are appropriate:
   (a) Intravenous diazepam
   (b) Intramuscular phenytoin
   (c) Measurement of blood glucose
   (d) Administration of 24% oxygen
   (e) Once the acute episode is over oral gabapentin should be commenced

133 Febrile convulsions:
   (a) Approximately 3% of children have at least one febrile convulsion
   (b) A prolonged convulsion can usually be terminated with rectal diazepam
   (c) Paracetamol is contraindicated in children who have febrile convulsion
   (d) Regular prophylaxis with phenobarbitone reduces the likelihood of adult epilepsy
   (e) Children with recurrent febrile convulsions should take prophylactic penicillin

134 In acute migraine the following are correct:
   (a) Paracetamol or aspirin is usually the treatment of choice
   (b) Metoclopramide may be effective due to its dopamine agonist action
   (c) Ergotamine may be given by the rectal route
   (d) Sumatriptan probably works through its $5HT_{1D}$-agonist properties
   (e) Pizotifen is effective when given by intramuscular injection during the acute episode

135 Sumatriptan:
   (a) Has a greater bioavailability after subcutaneous injection than oral administration
   (b) Is contraindicated in patients with ischemic heart disease
   (c) Causes a significant, but transient, pressor response
   (d) Should not be combined with ergotamine
   (e) Metabolism is inhibited by paracetamol

136 The following are used in the prophylaxis of migraine:
   (a) Sumatriptan
   (b) Ergotamine
   (c) Pizotifen
   (d) Propranolol
   (e) Methysergide

137 Halothane:

   (a) Has powerful analgesic properties
   (b) Warning signs of overdosage include bradycardia, hypotension and
       tachypnea
   (c) Is useful when quiet spontaneous respiration is required
   (d) Increases cerebral blood flow
   (e) Is contraindicated in children

138 Of halothane, enflurane and isoflurane:

   (a) Halothane is most likely to cause hepatic necrosis
   (b) Isoflurane is the least likely to cause cardiac dysrhythmias
   (c) Halothane is used if rapid recovery is important
   (d) Enflurane is the most potent anticonvulsant
   (e) Isoflurane is the agent of choice during neurosurgery

139 Nitrous oxide:

   (a) Has powerful anaigesic properties
   (b) Is a powerful muscle relaxant
   (c) After cessation of administration, diffusion hypoxia may occur
   (d) Is contraindicated if pethidine has been administered
   (e) Should not be premixed with oxygen

140 Propofol in comparison to sodium thiopentone:

   (a) Cannot be used for induction of anesthesia
   (b) Has a longer elimination half-life
   (c) Has no active metabolites
   (d) Is less irritant
   (e) Produces a more rapid "clear headed" recovery

141 The following agents are commonly used as premedication for anesthesia:

   (a) Hyoscine
   (b) Lorazepam
   (c) Papaveretum
   (d) Neostigmine
   (e) Ketamine

142 Atracurium:

   (a) Is a non-depolarizing muscle relaxant
   (b) Has histamine-blocking properties
   (c) May be used as a continuous infusion in intensive care to facilitate
       intermittent positive pressure ventilation
   (d) Is metabolized in the liver
   (e) Patients with reduced renal function show reduced elimination and
       prolonged neuromuscular blockade

137 (a) **False**   Halothane is a potent anesthetic but weak analgesic. It has a
    (b) **True**   low therapeutic index.
    (c) **True**
    (d) **True**
    (e) **False**

138 (a) **True**   Halothane rarely produces massive hepatic necrosis but
    (b) **True**   much more commonly produces subclinical hepatitis.
    (c) **False**   Enflurane and isoflurane are popular when multiple
    (d) **False**   anesthetics are used and rapid recovery is important.
    (e) **True**   Isoflurane is the least likely to cause dysrhythmias and has
    the least effect on cerebral blood flow.

139 (a) **True**   Nitrous oxide is commonly combined with volatile anesthetics
    (b) **False**   for its analgesic properties. Premixed nitrous oxide and
    (c) **True**   oxygen mixtures are used in obstetric practice and by
    (d) **False**   ambulance drivers.
    (e) **False**

140 (a) **False**   Sodium thiopentone, an ultra short-acting barbiturate is used
    (b) **False**   primarily as an induction agent. Propofol is used both for
    (c) **True**   induction, maintenance and anesthesia and sedation on
    (d) **True**   intensive care units.
    (e) **True**

141 (a) **True**   The chief aim of premedication is to allay anxiety in the
    (b) **True**   patient awaiting surgery. Inadequate premedication may lead
    (c) **True**   to the administration of larger doses of anesthetic than would
    (d) **False**   otherwise have been required resulting in delayed recovery.
    (e) **False**   Neostigmine, an anticholinesterase, may be used at the end
    of a procedure to reverse non-depolarizing muscle relaxants
    such as tubocurarine. Ketamine is a parenteral anesthetic
    which has a wide therapeutic index. Although it is a potent
    analgesic and sedative it can cause vivid unpleasant halluci-
    nations which may recur for months. It increases muscle tone
    and blood pressure. It is useful in major disasters for rapid,
    safe anaesthesia of trapped casualties to carry out procedures
    such as amputation.

142 (a) **True**   Atracurium has a rapid onset of action. It occasionally causes
    (b) **False**   histamine release leading to flushing of the face and chest,
    (c) **True**   hypotension and rarely bronchospasm. Continuous infusion is
    (d) **False**   popular in intensive care. It is inactivated spontaneously in the
    (e) **False**   plasma which is a valuable property in hepatic and renal
    failure.

143 The following would be suitable for postoperative analgesia in a patient with severe chronic obstructive airways disease with CO_2 rentention who has had an abdominoperineal resection:

   (a) Intramuscular morphine
   (b) Epidural block with bupivacaine
   (c) Rectal diclofenac
   (d) Intramuscular diclofenac
   (e) Oral co-proxamol

144 The following are included in the management of malignant hyperthermia due to volatile anesthetics or suxamethonium:

   (a) Discontinuation of anesthetic
   (b) 100% oxygen
   (c) Intravenous dantrolene
   (d) Correction of acidosis and hyperkalemia
   (e) Cooling

145 Lignocaine, a local anesthetic:

   (a) Prevents the rapid inflow of sodium ions which is the ionic basis of the action potential
   (b) Causes vasoconstriction
   (c) Is not absorbed from the urethra
   (d) Can be combined with adrenaline for digital "ring" blocks
   (e) Has a shorter duration of action than bupivacaine

146 The following drugs are correctly paired with their putative site(s) of action:

   (a) Non-steroidal anti-inflammatory drugs – at the site of injury, by interfering with the chemical mediators involved in nociception
   (b) Paracetamol – peripheral inhibition of cyclo-oxygenase
   (c) Lignocaine – block of transmission in peripheral nerves
   (d) Opioids – modification of transmission at the dorsal horn
   (e) Opioids – interference with central appreciation of pain and inhibition of emotional concomitants

147 Aspirin:

   (a) Inhibits cyclo-oxygenase irreversibly
   (b) Produces its major analgesic and anti-inflammatory effects by inhibition of prostaglandin E_2 and prostacyclin biosynthesis
   (c) Impairs color vision
   (d) Acts on the hypothalamus to reduce body temperature
   (e) Chronic use is associated with iron deficiency anemia

148 Adverse effects associated with salicylates include:

   (a) Claudication
   (b) Bronchoconstriction
   (c) Systemic lupus erythematosus
   (d) Hepatitis
   (e) Reye's syndrome

143 (a) **False**   Opioids may cause fatal respiratory depression. Even
    (b) **True**   epidural opioids can depress respiration and in this situation
    (c) **False**   epidural "local" anesthesia and intramuscular non-steroidal
    (d) **True**   anti-inflammatory drugs are preferred.
    (e) **False**

144 (a) **True**   Malignant hyperthermia is a rare but potentially lethal compli-
    (b) **True**   cation of anesthesia. It consists of a rapid increase in body
    (c) **True**   temperature accompanied by tachycardia and generalized
    (d) **True**   muscle spasm. Severe acidosis and hyperkalemia occur.
    (e) **True**   Dantrolene reverses the muscle spasm.

145 (a) **True**   Small unmyelinated fibers are depressed first hence the order
    (b) **False**   of loss of function is pain, temperature, touch, proprioception
    (c) **False**   and motor function. Lignocaine does not affect vascular
    (d) **False**   smooth muscle but is available with adrenaline, a vasocon-
    (e) **True**   strictor which prolongs its local effect. This combination may
                       cause vasospasm and severe digital ischemia if used for a
                       "ring" block hence the combination is contraindicated in this
                       situation. Bupivacaine is a long-acting local anesthetic which
                       is often used for peripheral nerve, plexus, epidural and spinal
                       anesthesia. Toxicity incudes ventricular fibrillation.

146 (a) **True**   Paracetamol probably produces its analgesic effect by central
    (b) **False**   inhibition of cyclo-oxygenase. It is antipyretic but not anti-
    (c) **True**   inflammatory.
    (d) **True**
    (e) **True**

147 (a) **True**   Gastric irritation is reduced by taking the drug after food.
    (b) **True**
    (c) **False**
    (d) **True**
    (e) **True**

148 (a) **False**   The commonest adverse effect associated with salicylates is
    (b) **True**   dyspepsia. Chronic blood loss from the stomach may be
    (c) **False**   asymptomatic. Salicylism which is associated with high blood
    (d) **True**   concentrations consists of tinnitus, deafness, nausea, vomiting
    (e) **True**   and occasionally abdominal pain and flushing.

149 Ibuprofen:

    (a) Is a reversible cyclo-oxygenase inhibitor
    (b) Has analgesic properties
    (c) Has antipyretic properties
    (d) Has anti-inflammatory properties
    (e) Can cause renal impairment

150 Nefopam:

    (a) Is associated with gastrointestinal hemorrhage
    (b) Causes meiosis
    (c) Causes more respiratory depression than morphine
    (d) Potentiates the arrhythmogenic effect of halothane anesthesia
    (e) Is contraindicated in epilepsy

151 Co-proxamol contains:

    (a) Aspirin
    (b) Paracetamol
    (c) Dextropropoxyphene
    (d) Caffeine
    (e) Promethazine

152 Morphine:

    (a) Acts as an agonist at opioid receptors (especially μ) in the brain and spinal cord
    (b) Causes pupillary constriction by stimulation of the Edinger–Westphal nucleus in the mid-brain
    (c) Acts as an antihistamine
    (d) Is subject to presystemic metabolism
    (e) Stimulates the chemoreceptor trigger zone

153 The following are particulalry sensitive to the pharmacological actions of morphine:

    (a) Young children
    (b) The elderly
    (c) Patients with hepatic failure
    (d) Patients with renal failure
    (e) Patients with hyperthyroidism

154 Morphine causes:

    (a) Diarrhea
    (b) Increased intrabiliary pressure
    (c) Histamine release
    (d) Reduced sensitivity of the respiratory center to carbon dioxide
    (e) Vasoconstriction

149 (a) True
(b) True
(c) True
(d) True
(e) True

Ibuprofen is a non-steroidal anti-inflammatory drug which is available without prescription. The side effects are those of all the NSAIDs of which gastrointestinal irritation is the most common.

150 (a) False
(b) False
(c) False
(d) True
(e) True

Nefopam is chemically and pharmacologically unrelated to opioids and NSAIDs. It is used for moderately severe pain. It can cause fatal hypertension if prescribed during or within 2 weeks of cessation of non-selective MAO inhibitor treatment.

151 (a) False
(b) True
(c) True
(d) False
(e) False

Co-proxamol, a compound analgesic of dextropropoxyphene and paracetamol is widely prescribed. It is dangerous in over-dose (see *CPT*, Chapter 50). When taking a drug history one must be aware that many over-the-counter remedies contain a surprising mixture of pharmacologically active agents, although often in almost "homeopathic" quantities.

152 (a) True
(b) True
(c) False
(d) True
(e) True

– The most important use of morphine is pain relief

153 (a) True
(b) True
(c) True
(d) True
(e) False

Patients with decreased respiratory reserve and myxedema are also more senstive.

154 (a) False
(b) True
(c) True
(d) True
(e) False

Morphine increases smooth muscle tone throughout the gastrointestinal tract and in addition reduces peristalsis through an action on the receptors in the ganglion plexus in the gut wall which results in constipation.

155 Diamorphine:

    (a) Is metabolized to morphine and 6-acetylmorphine
    (b) Has a half-life after intravenous injection of approximately 3 minutes
    (c) Has a less rapid clinical effect than morphine
    (d) Is contraindicated in left ventricular failure
    (e) Is antagonized by naloxone

156 Pethidine:

    (a) Is more potent than morphine
    (b) Does not cause respiratory depression
    (c) Always causes pupillary constriction at analgesic doses
    (d) Suppresses cough at analgesic doses
    (e) Reduces the activity of the pregnant term uterus

157 Codeine:

    (a) Is a metabolite of morphine
    (b) Has a plasma half-life of approximately 12 hours
    (c) Is not antagonized by naloxone
    (d) Is used as a cough suppressant
    (e) Causes constipation

158 Buprenorphine:

    (a) Is a partial agonist on opioid receptors
    (b) Occupies a much larger fraction of opioid receptors to produce its analgesic effect than does morphine
    (c) Should only be used to treat acute pain
    (d) Is subject to prescription requirements under the Misuse of Drugs Act
    (e) May be administered sublingually

159 Naloxone:

    (a) Binds to opioid μ receptors
    (b) Acts as a partial opioid agonist
    (c) Has little effect on a healthy person who has not taken opioid drugs
    (d) Has an elimination half-life of approximately 12 hours
    (e) Is contraindicated in young children

155 **(a) True**   Diamorphine is diacetylmorphine. Its actions are similar to
      (b) True   those of morphine but is more potent as an analgesic when
      (c) False   given by injection. It is more soluble than morphine.
      (d) False   Diamorphine and 6-acetylmorphine enter the brain more
      (e) True   rapidly than morphine.

156 **(a) False**   Pethidine causes similar respiratory depression and vomiting
      (b) False   to morphine but does not release histamine or suppress
      (c) False   cough and only uncommonly produces pupillary constriction to
      (d) False   the same extent as morphine.
      (e) False

157 **(a) False**   Morphine is a metabolite of codeine. Codeine is used as an
      (b) False   analgesic, cough suppressant and antidiarrheal agent. The
      (c) False   plasma half-life is 3–4 hours.
      (d) True
      (e) True

158 **(a) True**   In common with other partial agonists buprenorphine occupies
      (b) True   a much larger fraction of the receptors to produce its
      (c) False   analgesic effect than does a full agonist. Consequently it can
      (d) True   precipitate pain and cause withdrawal symptoms in patients
      (e) True   who have received other opioids and relatively much larger
                   doses of naloxone are required to displace it from receptors
                   in overdosage compared to a full agonist.

159 **(a) True**   Naxolone is a pure competitive antagonist. It has a half-life of
      (b) False   1 hour which is less than many opioids.
      (c) True
      (d) False
      (e) False

3 MUSCULOSKELETAL SYSTEM

160 Ibuprofen:

    (a) Inhibits the enzyme cyclo-oxygenase irreversibly

    (b) Inhibits leukotriene biosynthesis

    (c) Is a more potent anti-inflammatory agent than indomethacin

    (d) May precipitate asthma

    (e) Reduces lithium clearance

161 Sulindac:

    (a) Is a non-steroidal anti-inflammatory drug

    (b) Is a pro-drug

    (c) Is ineffective in gout

    (d) Is contraindicated in hypertension

    (e) Is less likely to cause gastritis than paracetamol

162 The following drugs inhibit cyclo-oxygenase:

    (a) Diclofenac

    (b) Gold salts

    (c) Penicillamine

    (d) Chloroquine

    (e) Methotrexate

163 Gold salts when used in the treatment of progressive rheumatoid arthritis

    (a) Are usually administered daily by intravenous injection

    (b) If effective, benefit should be observed after the first week of treatment

    (c) About 75% of patients show an objective improvement

    (d) Rashes are an indication to stop treatment

    (e) If stomatitis occurs this suggests the possibility of neutropenia

164 Penicillamine is used in the management of:

    (a) Rheumatoid arthritis

    (b) Systemic lupus erythematosus (SLE)

    (c) Wilson's disease

    (d) Cystinuria

    (e) Lead poisoning

165 Adverse effects associated with penicillamine include:

    (a) Thrombocytopenia

    (b) Leukopenia

    (c) Immune complex glomerulonephritis

    (d) Taste loss

    (e) Myasthenia gravis

160 (a) **False**   All NSAIDs inhibit cyclo-oxygenase reversibly except aspirin.
    (b) **False**   All have analgesic and anti-inflammatory properties.
    (c) **False**   Inhibition of prostaglandin E_2 biosynthesis is associated with
    (d) **True**   increased leukotriene B_4 biosynthesis.
    (e) **True**

161 (a) **True**   Sulindac is a NSAID which is relatively "renal sparing". It acts
    (b) **True**   through an active sulfide metabolite which in the kidney is
    (c) **False**   converted back into the inactive sulfone.
    (d) **False**
    (e) **False**

162 (a) **True**   Several drugs are not analgesic and do not inhibit cyclo-
    (b) **False**   oxygenase but do suppress the inflammatory process in
    (c) **False**   rheumatoid arthritis. They only have a part to play in patients
    (d) **False**   with progressive disease.
    (e) **False**

163 (a) **False**   Gold (as sodium aurothiomalate) is usually administered as
    (b) **False**   weekly intramuscular injections or by mouth daily. Benefit is
    (c) **True**   not anticipated for at least 6 weeks. Blood dyscrasias and
    (d) **True**   glomerular injury (nephrotic syndrome) occur and monitoring
    (e) **True**   of blood counts and urine is performed monthly. Rashes may
    progress to exfoliation.

164 (a) **True**   Penicillamine, a breakdown product of penicillin, is given by
    (b) **False**   mouth. In rheumatoid arthritis clinical improvement is
    (c) **True**   anticipated only after 6–12 weeks. It is contraindicated in SLE.
    (d) **True**
    (e) **True**

165 (a) **True**   The toxicity of penicillamine is such that it should only be
    (b) **True**   used by clinicians with experience of the drug and with
    (c) **True**   meticulous patient monitoring.
    (d) **True**
    (e) **True**

166 The following are likely to be effective in the treatment of an acute episode of gout:

  (a) Indomethacin
  (b) Naproxen
  (c) Allopurinol
  (d) Probenecid
  (e) Colchicine

167 The following may cause hyperuricemia:

  (a) Sulfinpyrazone
  (b) Cytotoxic drugs in the treatment of leukemia
  (c) Bendrofluazide
  (d) Low doses of salicylates
  (e) Bezafibrate

168 Allopurinol:

  (a) Inhibits xanthine oxidase
  (b) May provoke acute gout
  (c) Is contraindicated in renal failure
  (d) Should not be prescribed with a NSAID
  (e) Inactivates azathioprine

166 **(a) True**   Acute gout is treated by anti-inflammatory analgesic agents.
     (b) True   Colchicine is an alternative in those unable to tolerate NSAIDs
     (c) False   but commonly causes diarrhea.
     (d) False
     (e) True

167 **(a) False**   Uric acid is the end product of purine metabolism in humans,
     (b) True   and gives rise to problems because of its limited solubility.
     (c) True   Diuretics, low dose salicylates and pyrazinamide
     (d) True   inhibit tubular excretion of uric acid.
     (e) False

168 **(a) True**   Allopurinol is used as long-term medication to treat patients
     (b) True   with recurrent gout. By inhibiting xanthine oxidase it
     (c) False   decreases uric acid production. It potentiates azathioprine
     (d) False   by blocking inactivation of its active metabolite 6-mercaptop
     (e) False   urine.

4 CARDIOVASCULAR SYSTEM

169 Cholestyramine:

  (a) Causes a fall in plasma cholesterol
  (b) Increases fecal excretion of bile acids
  (c) Reduces absorption of folic acid
  (d) Causes diarrhea in diabetic autonomic neuropathy
  (e) Reduces pruritus in incomplete biliary obstruction

170 Bezafibrate:

  (a) Lowers plasma triglyceride
  (b) Is ineffective post-cholecystectomy
  (c) Inhibits lipoprotein lipase
  (d) Is indicated in alcohol-induced hyperlipidemia
  (e) Potentiates the effects of warfarin

171 Simvastatin, an HMGCoA reductase inhibitor:

  (a) Lowers low density liporotein (LDL) cholesterol
  (b) Is particularly useful in heterozygous familial hypercholesterolemia
  (c) Acts locally on HMGCoA reductase in the intestine
  (d) Is associated with rhabdomyolysis
  (e) Is ineffective if prescribed with a bile acid binding resin

172 Probucol:

  (a) Lowers plasma LDL cholesterol
  (b) Lowers plasma high density lipoprotein (HDL) cholesterol
  (c) Lowers plasma triglyceride
  (d) Causes regression of tendon xanthomata of patients with familial hypercholesterolemia
  (e) Is associated with prolongation of the QT interval of the ECG

173 The following can cause hypertension:

  (a) Corticosteroid therapy
  (b) Oral contraception
  (c) Alcohol withdrawal
  (d) Opioid withdrawal
  (e) Ergotamine

174 Thiazide diuretics when used in the management of uncomplicated essential hypertension:

  (a) Reduce the risk of stroke
  (b) Are natriuretic
  (c) Potassium supplements are usually required
  (d) Reduce plasma renin
  (e) Are associated with impotence

169 (a) **True**   The anion exchange resins cholestyramine and colestipol are
     (b) **True**   not absorbed into the systemic circulation and bind bile acids
     (c) **False**   in the gut lumen inhibiting reabsorption of bile salts and
     (d) **False**   cholesterol. Cholestyramine causes malabsorption of fat-
     (e) **True**   soluble vitamins, and is used to treat pruritus in patients with
                      incomplete biliary obstruction.

170 (a) **True**   The fibrates stimulate lipoprotein lipase and reduce plasma
     (b) **False**   triglyceride. They can cause myositis which is more common
     (c) **False**   in alcoholics and in patients on concurrent HMGCoA
     (d) **False**   reductase inhibitors.
     (e) **True**

171 (a) **True**   HMGCoA reductase is the rate-limiting step in cholesterol
     (b) **True**   biosynthesis from acetate. HMGCoA inhibitors are ineffective
     (c) **False**   in rare patients with homozygous familial hypercholesterolemia
     (d) **True**   because they cannot make LDL-receptors.
     (e) **False**

172 (a) **True**   Probucol stimulates non-receptor-mediated LDL catabolism. It
     (b) **True**   is a powerful antioxidant but may cause ventricular
     (c) **False**   tachycardia.
     (d) **True**
     (e) **True**

173 (a) **True**   Although hypertension is usually "essential" (i.e. idiopathic)
     (b) **True**   the possibility of secondary hypertension must always be
     (c) **True**   considered. Equally important is the confirmation or rejection
     (d) **True**   of persistent hypertention by repeated measures (blood
     (e) **True**   pressure is very variable) and the identification of other
                      treatable risk factors such as diabetes, smoking, hypercholes
                      terolemia and obesity.

174 (a) **True**   Thiazide diuretics (e.g. bendrofluazide, hydrochlorthiazide)
     (b) **True**   remain the logical first choice for treating patients with mild
     (c) **False**   hypertension unless contraindicated by some co-existant
     (d) **False**   disease and are also valuable in patients with more severe
     (e) **True**   hypertension in combination with other therapy.

175 Thiazide diuretics are associated with:

   (a) Purpura
   (b) Hyperuricemia
   (c) Hyperglycemia
   (d) Hypercalcemia
   (e) Hypercholesterolemia

176 β-adrenoceptor antagonists:

   (a) Reduce the risk of stroke in hypertension
   (b) Reduce the risk of myocardial infarction in hypertension
   (c) Improve performance of sprinters
   (d) The antihypertensive effect is antagonized by NSAIDs
   (e) May be effectively combined with thiazide diuretics in reducing a raised blood pressure

177 The following drugs when used as monotherapy in the management of hypertension are likely to be less effective in Afro-Caribbeans than in Caucasians:

   (a) Atenolol
   (b) Enalapril
   (c) Bendrofluazide
   (d) Nifedipine
   (e) Doxazosin

178 β-adrenoceptor antagonists are contraindicated in:

   (a) Asthma
   (b) Heart failure
   (c) Second degree heart block
   (d) Dissecting thoracic aneurysm
   (e) Migraine

179 Captopril, an angiotensin-converting enzyme (ACE) inhibitor:

   (a) Reduces concentrations of angiotensin II
   (b) Increases concentrations of bradykinin
   (c) Increases noradrenaline release from sympathetic nerve terminals
   (d) Increases aldosterone secretion
   (e) Blocks angiotensin II receptors

180 Captopril is contraindicated in:

   (a) Left ventricular failure
   (b) Asthma
   (c) Bilateral renal artery stenosis
   (d) Pregnancy
   (e) Diabetic nephropathy

181 Nifedipine, a dihydropyridine calcium channel blocker:

   (a) Dilates veins more than arteries
   (b) Can be combined with β-blockers in the management of hypertension
   (c) Increases plasma calcium concentration
   (d) Is contraindicated in diabetes mellitus
   (e) Raises the plasma concentration of cholesterol

175 (a) True
    (b) True
    (c) True
    (d) True
    (e) True

Thiazide diuretics are generally well tolerated. Treatment should be initated with a low dose (e.g. 2.5 mg bendro-fluazide). Higher doses increase the incidence of adverse effects relatively more than efficacy.

176 (a) True
    (b) True
    (c) False
    (d) True
    (e) True

The relatively cardioselective β_1-adrenoreceptor antagonists, atenolol and metoprolol, are widely used to treat hypertension in the UK. They are particularly valuable in patients with angina or who have survived a myocardial infarction.

177 (a) True
    (b) True
    (c) False
    (d) False
    (e) False

Afro-Caribbean patients are less likely to have high circulating renin levels hence β-blockers and ACE inhibitors are less likely to be effective. This difference is statistical and based on large populations and both ACE inhibitors and β-blockers can be effective in Afro-Caribbean patients but a thiazide is usually the antihypertensive of first choice.

178 (a) True
    (b) True
    (c) True
    (d) False
    (d) False

In addition to asthma, heart failure and heart block, β-blockers aggravate peripheral vascular disease and vasospasm and mask the symptoms of hypoglycemia. In some individuals they cause fatigue and hallucinations. They reduce the somatic symptoms of anxiety.

179 (a) True
    (b) True
    (c) False
    (d) False
    (e) False

ACE inhibitors inhibit the conversion of inactive angiotensin I to active angiotensin II, a powerful vasoconstrictor, and also inhibit the breakdown of the vasodilator peptides such as bradykinin. This latter effect may cause cough.

180 (a) False
    (b) False
    (c) True
    (d) True
    (e) False

Plasma creatinine and potassium should be monitored before and during the early weeks of therapy with ACE inhibitors and the possibilty of bilateral renal artery stenosis (one of the few correctable causes of hypertension) considered if there is a marked rise in creatinine. Glomerular filtration in these patients is dependent on angiotensin-II mediated efferent arteriolar vasoconstriction.

181 (a) False
    (b) True
    (c) False
    (d) False
    (e) False

Nifedipine is used in the management of Raynaud's syndrome, hypertension and angina.

182 Nifedipine in comparison to verapamil is more likely to:

  (a) Worsen angina
  (b) Cause ankle swelling unresponsive to diuretics
  (c) Have negative inotropic effects
  (d) Cause flushing and headache
  (e) Cause constipation

183 Prazosin:

  (a) Is a selective reversible α_1-blocker
  (b) Should always be prescribed with a β-blocker to prevent reflex tachycardia
  (c) Is associated with first dose hypotension
  (d) Reduces plasma LDL cholesterol
  (e) Has a shorter half-life than doxazosin

184 Sodium nitroprusside:

  (a) Is administered by intravenous infusion
  (b) Prolonged administration can lead to cyanide poisoning
  (c) Has a half-life of about 1 week
  (d) Reduces cardiac "pre-load"
  (e) Reduces cardiac "afterload"

185 Methyldopa:

  (a) Causes central α_2-agonist effects
  (b) Causes drowsiness and fatigue
  (c) Pyrexia is an adverse effect
  (d) Is associated with Coombs positive hemolytic anemia
  (e) A single missed dose can cause profound rebound hypertension

186 The following hypotensive combinations are rational when a single drug has not been effective in treating essential hypertension:

  (a) Thiazide and atenolol
  (b) Thiazide and captopril in an asthmatic
  (c) Amiloride and captopril in an asthmatic who has gout
  (d) Nifedipine and verapamil in a man who has had thiazide-induced impotence and captopril-induced rash
  (e) Enalapril and doxazosin in a man with prostatism

187 The following drug effects have been correctly paired with the named drug:

  (a) Hydralazine – drug-induced SLE
  (b) Minoxidil – hirsutism
  (c) Captopril – first dose hypotension
  (d) Atenolol – tremor
  (e) Clonidine – bronchospasm

182 **(a) True**   Nifedipine, unlike verapamil, has no effect on the conducting
      (b) True   system of the heart. In the occasional patient it can worsen
      (c) False   angina due to a reflex tachycardia whilst verapamil causes a
      (d) True   a bradycardia. Both drugs are effective arterial dilators.
      (e) False   Verapamil is a much more potent negative inotrope.

183 **(a) True**   Non-specific α-blockers such as phenoxybenzamine cause
      (b) False   profound postural hypotension and reflex tachycardia.
      (c) True   Prazosin does not block presynaptic α_2-receptors that are
      (d) True   normally stimulated by released noradrenaline and which
      (e) True   inhibit further transmitter release. This is a negative feedback
                   pathway hence there is little reflex tachycardia with prazosin
                   although first dose hypotension is a problem.

184 **(a) True**   Sodium nitroprusside is valuable in treating hypertensive
      (b) True   encephalopathy and in the management of certain types of
      (c) False   "shock" when it is combined with positive inotropes.
      (d) True   Continuous BP monitoring is essential as it causes profound
      (e) True   hypotension. It has a half-life of seconds.

185 **(a) True**   Although generally safe and not contraindicated in asthma
      (b) True   and pregnancy, methyldopa is often poorly tolerated.
      (c) True   Drowsiness and fatigue may be intolerable when used
      (d) True   chronically. It is a well recognized (but uncommon) cause of
      (e) False   drug fever and Coombs positive hemolytic anemia.

186 **(a) True**   Most hypertensive patients are successfully treated with a
      (b) True   single drug. Diuretics worsen symptoms of bladder neck
      (c) False   obstruction, whereas α_1 antagonists improve such symptoms
      (d) False   as well as synergizing with ACE inhibitors.
      (e) True

187 **(a) True**   – More common in slow acetylators
      (b) True   – Fluid retention is also a problem
      (c) True   – Worse if on diuretics
      (d) False
      (e) False   – Rebound hypertension, dry mouth, depression and sedation are
                   the main adverse effects

188 The following hypotensive drugs have a potentially deleterious effect on lipid profile:

(a) Thiazide diuretics
(b) β-blockers
(c) Captopril
(d) Nifedipine
(e) Doxazosin

189 The following drugs are considered to have particular value for the indication named:

(a) Hypertension in a diabetic with albuminuria – captopril
(b) Hypertension and ischemic heart disease in a patient with asthma – nifedipine
(c) Acute aortic dissection – sodium nitroprusside
(d) Hypertension in a professional soccer player – atenolol
(e) Imminent eclampsia – hydralazine

190 Management of acute myocardial infarction should usually include (unless contraindicated):

(a) 24% oxygen
(b) Intravenous opiate with an antiemetic
(c) Aspirin
(d) A fibrinolytic drug (e.g. streptokinase)
(e) Lignocaine

191 The management of unstable angina usually includes:

(a) Aspirin
(b) Glyceryl trinitrate
(c) Intravenous heparin
(d) Dipyridamole
(e) α-adrenoceptor antagonist

192 Glyceryl trinitrate (GTN):

(a) Relaxes vascular smooth muscle
(b) Is associated with tolerance more commonly with transdermal GTN patches than sublingual GTN
(c) Is volatile
(d) Is relatively more selective for arteriolar than for venous smooth muscle
(e) May relieve the pain of esophageal spasm

193 β-adrenoceptor antagonists:

(a) Increase cardiac tissue cyclic adenosine monophosphate (cAMP)
(b) Competitively antagonize the β-receptor mediated effects of adrenaline and noradrenaline
(c) Non-competitively antagonize several of the actions of thyroxine
(d) Decrease peripheral vascular resistance
(e) Reduce renin secretion

188 (a) **True**　　　The potentially deleterious effects on lipid profile are of
　　　(b) **True**　　　unproven clinical significance to date.
　　　(c) **False**
　　　(d) **False**
　　　(e) **False**

189 (a) **True**　　　The choice of hypotensive drug must be individually
　　　(b) **True**　　　tailored to the patient. The first line drugs in uncomplicated
　　　(c) **True**　　　hypertension remain a thiazide or a β-blocker in patients
　　　(d) **False**　　　without contraindications.
　　　(e) **True**

190 (a) **False**　　　The highest concentration of oxygen available should be
　　　(b) **True**　　　used unless there is coincident pulmonary disease with
　　　(c) **True**　　　CO_2 retention. Aspirin and thrombolytic therapy have an
　　　(d) **True**　　　additive beneficial effect on reduction of infarct size and
　　　(e) **False**　　　improvement in survival.

191 (a) **True**　　　Patients with unstable angina require urgent antiplatelet
　　　(b) **True**　　　therapy (aspirin) and urgent admission.
　　　(c) **True**
　　　(d) **False**
　　　(e) **False**

192 (a) **True**　　　GTN is generally best used as acute prophylaxis (i.e.
　　　(b) **True**　　　immediately before undertaking strenuous activity). The
　　　(c) **True**　　　spray has a longer "shelf-life" but is more expensive than
　　　(d) **False**　　　the sublingual GTN. GTN is subject to extensive
　　　(e) **True**　　　presystemic metabolism if swallowed. Longer acting oral
　　　　　　　　　　　nitrates (e.g. isosorbide mononitrate) are effective as
　　　　　　　　　　　regular prophylactic therapy.

193 (a) **False**　　　β-Blockers slow the heart, are negatively inotropic and
　　　(b) **True**　　　reduce arterial blood pressure, are anti-arrhythmic,
　　　(c) **True**　　　increase peripheral vascular resistance, reduce plasma
　　　(d) **False**　　　renin activity and predispose to bronchoconstriction.
　　　(e) **True**

194 β-Adrenoceptor antagonists should be avoided in:
- (a) Coronary artery spasm
- (b) Second degree heart block
- (c) Asthma well controlled with salbutamol
- (d) Aortic aneurysm
- (e) Raynaud's disease

195 Nifedipine is used:
- (a) For prophylaxis of angina
- (b) To treat hypertension
- (c) To treat supraventricular tachycardia
- (d) To prevent cerebral vasospasm following subarachnoid hemorrhage
- (e) To treat coronary artery spasm

196 A calcium channel blocker (e.g. nifedipine) is preferred to a β-blocker (e.g. atenolol) to treat angina in patients who also have:
- (a) Chronic bronchitis
- (b) Peripheral vascular disease
- (c) Heart block
- (d) Diabetes
- (e) Anxiety

197 Aspirin:
- (a) Reduces the risk of stroke in patients with transient ischemic attacks
- (b) Predisposes to peptic ulceration
- (c) Irreversibly inhibits fatty acid cyclo-oxygenase
- (d) Has no effect on bleeding time
- (e) Needs to be given twice daily to prevent platelet cyclo-oxygenase resynthesis within the dose interval

198 Streptokinase:
- (a) Is derived from streptococci
- (b) Reduces the acute mortality of myocardial infarction only if administered within 4 hours of the onset of chest pain
- (c) Is contraindicated if the patient is taking regular non-steroidal anti-Inflammatory drug therapy
- (d) Is administered by intravenous infusion
- (e) Should not be given to patients over the age of 60 years

199 Alteplase:
- (a) Is a prodrug that liberates streptokinase
- (b) Heparin must not be administered within 24 hours of alteplase infusion
- (c) Should only be administered if pulmonary artery pressure can be measured
- (d) Is administered via the intramuscular route
- (e) Is contraindicated if aspirin has been administered in the last 24 hours

194 **(a) True** – Due to unopposed α-adrenoceptor vasoconstriction
(b) True – Unless the patient is already paced
(c) True – Asthma is an absolute contraindication
(d) False – β-blockers are helpful in reducing blood pressure and the risk of dissection
(e) True – Also may aggravate claudication

195 **(a) True** Nifedipine is also used to treat Raynaud's disease. Verapamil
(b) True is used to treat supraventricular tachycardia and nimodipine
(c) False to prevent cerebral vasospasm.
(d) False
(e) True

196 **(a) True** The commonest side effects of nifedipine are flushing and
(b) True headache.
(c) True
(d) True
(e) False

197 **(a) True** Thromboxane (TX) A_2 is the main cyclo-oxygenase product of
(b) True activated platelets and is proaggregatory and a
(c) True vasoconstrictor.
(d) False
(e) False

198 **(a) True** Streptokinase combines with plasminogen to form an
(b) False activator complex that converts remaining free plasminogen
(c) False to plasmin which dissolves fibrin. The potential benefit
(d) True lessens with delay but the value of treatment within 24 hours
(e) False is well established.

199 **(a) False** Alteplase is a direct-acting plasminogen activator. Immediate
(b) False heparin following alteplase is necessary to prevent
(c) False re-occlusion.
(d) False
(e) False

200 The following are relative contraindications to the use of streptokinase in acute myocardial infarction:

(a) Therapy with anistreplase from 5 days to 12 months previously
(b) Stroke due to cerebral thrombosis in the last 6 months
(c) Concurrent hormone replacement therapy for menopausal symptoms
(d) Pulmonary disease with cavitation
(e) Diabetic retinopathy

201 Heparin:

(a) Binds to antithrombin III
(b) Inhibits the action of thrombin
(c) Is monitored in the laboratory by measurement of activated partial thromboplastin time (APTT)
(d) Is less effective in patients with inherited or acquired deficiency of antithrombin III
(e) Is reversed by protamine sulfate

202 Heparin prophylaxis to prevent deep vein thrombosis/pulmonary embolism in major surgery:

(a) Must be started 1 week before surgery
(b) Is via twice daily intramuscular heparin
(c) Is more likely to be of value in an obese man of 50 than in a slim man of 30
(d) Low molecular weight heparin is an alternative to standard heparin
(e) Concomitant antibiotics are contraindicated

203 The following are recognized adverse effects of heparin therapy:

(a) Osteoporosis
(b) Alopecia
(c) Thrombocytopenia
(d) Diarrhea
(e) Fetal cleft palate

204 The following statements are correct:

(a) In the management of pulmonary embolism heparin is normally administered as an intravenous bolus followed by a continuous infusion
(b) Prophylactic subcutaneous heparin should be monitored by measurement of prothrombin time
(c) Heparin does not affect the thrombin time
(d) Heparin exhibits dose-dependent pharmacokinetics
(e) Immune thrombocytopenia is less common with low molecular weight heparin

200 **(a) True**   Immune reactions are important with streptokinase and
      (b) True   its prodrug anistreplase. It seems unlikely that mild
      (c) False   infections such as sore throats reduce its efficacy.
      (d) True   "Recent" dental extraction is considered a contraindication.
      (e) True

201 **(a) True**   Heparin binds to antithrombin III, the naturally occurring
      (b) True   inhibitor of thrombin and of the other serine proteases
      (c) True   (factors IXa, Xa and XIa), enormously potentiating its
      (d) True   inhibitory action.
      (e) True

202 **(a) False**   Prophylactic subcutaneous heparin reduces the risk of
      (b) False   thromboembolism associated with major surgery. A lower
      (c) True   concentration of heparin is required to inhibit factor Xa early
      (d) True   in the cascade than is needed to antagonize the actions
      (e) False   of thrombin and this provides the rationale for the use of low
                 dose heparin in prophylaxis. The benefit normally outweighs
                 the increased risk of bleeding in major orthopedic surgery.

203 **(a) True**   The commonest adverse effect is bleeding. This can be
      (b) True   treated by stopping the infusion (if relevant) local
      (c) True   compression, protamine sulfate and if severe and
      (d) False   continues in spite of the above, fresh frozen plasma.
      (e) False

204 **(a) True**   Owing to its short half-life (0.5–2.5 hours), dose-dependent
      (b) False   kinetics and wide interindividual variation intravenous heparin
      (c) False   is ideally administered as an infusion with monitoring of APTT.
      (d) True   Low molecular weight heparin (LMWH) is a more specific
      (e) True   anticoagulant which is used prophylactically at low doses and
                 occasionally in patients who have heparin-induced immune
                 thrombocytopenia. At normal doses LMWH does not prolong
                 APTT and is monitored by factor Xa assay. Although effective,
                 LMWH is expensive.

205 Warfarin:

(a) Prevents the hepatic synthesis of the vitamin-K dependent coagulation factors II, VII, IX and X
(b) Is structurally closely related to vitamin K
(c) Should initially be given as a subcutaneous loading dose
(d) During life-threatening bleeding can be reversed by vitamin K and factor IX concentrate
(e) Anticoagulant effect is monitored by measurement of the prothrombin time/INR (international normalized ratio)

206 The following are relative contraindications to warfarin therapy:

(a) First trimester of pregnancy
(b) Prosthetic heart valves
(c) Space-occupying CNS lesion
(d) Concurrent digoxin therapy
(e) G6PD deficiency

207 The following drugs inhibit the metabolism of warfarin:

(a) Cimetidine
(b) Amiodarone
(c) Dextropropoxyphene
(d) Carbamazepine
(e) The oral contraceptive

208 The following inhibit platelet activation and/or aggregation:

(a) Warfarin
(b) Heparin
(c) Thromboxane A_2
(d) Prostacyclin (epoprostenol)
(e) Dipyridamole

209 Prostacyclin (epoprostenol):

(a) Relaxes pulmonary and systemic vasculature
(b) Is the principal endogenous prostaglandin of large- and medium-sized blood vessels
(c) Is an effective anticoagulant
(d) Is contraindicated in hemodialysis
(e) Increases diastolic pressure

210 The principal beneficial effect in heart failure of the following drugs is to reduce preload (left ventricular filling pressure):

(a) Digoxin
(b) Frusemide
(c) Dobutamine
(d) GTN
(e) Sodium nitroprusside

205 (a) True   Warfarin is the most commonly prescribed oral anticoagulant.
    (b) True   It usually takes at least 3 days to achieve adequate anti-
    (c) False   coagulation. If more rapid action is required intravenous
    (d) True   heparin and oral warfarin are used until the INR is in the
    (e) True   usual therapeutic range (2–3 for most indications). Heparin
                  only influences the INR if the APTT > 2.5 the control. The
                  laboratory can allow for this by the *in vitro* addition of
                  protamine.

206 (a) True   Other contraindications include active bleeding, blood
    (b) False   dyscrasias with hemorrhagic diatheses, dissecting aneurysm
    (c) True   of the aorta and recent CNS surgery. Aspirin and warfarin
    (d) False   should not be used together routinely, although trials of low
    (e) False   dose combination therapy are in progress.

207 (a) True   Warfarin has a narrow therapeutic range and steep dose
    (b) True   response curve. The INR must be monitored to reduce both
    (c) True   the risk of bleeding and inadequate anticoagulation.
    (d) False
    (e) False

208 (a) False   Thromboxane A2 is synthesized by activated platelets and
    (b) True   acts on platelet receptors to cause further activation and
    (c) False   propagation of the aggregate. It also acts on vascular
    (d) True   smooth muscle to cause vasoconstriction. Heparin inhibits
    (e) True   thrombin, which is a platelet agonist, as well as causing
                  coagulation.

209 (a) True   Prostacyclin is used to prevent coagulation in extracorporeal
    (b) True   circuits. It causes flushing, headache, reduced diastolic
    (c) True   pressure, increased pulse pressure and usually a reflex
    (d) False   tachycardia. Occasionally vagally mediated bradycardia and
    (e) False   hypotension occur.

210 (a) False   The major influences on preload are blood volume and
    (b) True   capacitance vessel tone.
    (c) False
    (d) True
    (e) False

211 The following drugs aggravate heart failure:

    (a) Atenolol
    (b) Verapamil
    (c) Daunorubicin
    (d) Ibuprofen
    (e) Bendrofluazide

212 In acute pulmonary edema the following are usually appropriate:

    (a) Sublingual nifedipine
    (b) Lie the patient supine
    (c) Oxygen
    (d) Intravenous loop diuretic
    (e) Intravenous morphine

213 Intravenous frusemide:

    (a) Causes natriuresis
    (b) Causes kaliuresis
    (c) Has an indirect vasodilator effect
    (d) Diuresis begins 10–20 minutes after an intravenous dose
    (e) High doses are ototoxic

214 Angiotension-converting enzyme (ACE) inhibitors:

    (a) Are positive inotropes
    (b) Reduce afterload
    (c) Reduce preload
    (d) May cause cough
    (e) Should be given parenterally in acute heart failure

215 Dobutamine:

    (a) Is a sympathomimetic amine
    (b) Is predominantly a β_1-receptor agonist
    (c) Increases blood pressure via vasoconstriction
    (d) Should not be given concomitantly with intravenous dopamine
    (e) Increases myocardial oxygen consumption

216 Dopamine:

    (a) Inhibits phosphodiesterase
    (b) Is the biochemical precursor of noradrenaline
    (c) Is pro-arrhythmogenic
    (d) Is associated with convulsions
    (e) At low doses has a selective vasodilator effect on the renal vascular bed

217 The following drugs can cause sinus tachycardia:

    (a) Clonidine
    (b) Theophylline
    (c) Dobutamine
    (d) Amphetamine
    (e) Digoxin

211 (a) True
    (b) True
    (c) True
    (d) True
    (e) False

Negative inotropes, direct cardiac toxins (e.g. daunorubicin) and drugs that cause salt retention (e.g. NSAIDs) aggravate heart failure. *Excessive* tachycardia does not allow sufficient time for the ventricle to fill in diastole.

212 (a) False
    (b) False
    (c) True
    (d) True
    (e) True

In addition to helping relieve the acute anxiety and discomfort associated with acute pulmonary edema opioids dilate capacitance vessels.

213 (a) True
    (b) True
    (c) True
    (d) True
    (e) True

Loop diuretics inhibit $Na^+/K^+/2Cl^-$ cotransport in the thick ascending limb of Henlé's loop.

214 (a) False
    (b) True
    (c) True
    (d) True
    (e) False

ACE inhibitors are a major advance in the treatment of cardiac failure acting as arterial and venous vasodilators and prolonging survival.

215 (a) True
    (b) True
    (c) False
    (d) False
    (e) True

Dobutamine is a positive inotrope used predominantly in cardiogenic shock. Hypovolemia must be corrected before its use and measurement of pulmonary artery wedge pressure as an indicator of left sided filling pressure using a Swann–Ganz catheter is particularly helpful.

216 (a) False
    (b) True
    (c) True
    (d) False
    (e) True

Low dose dopamine increases renal blood flow. In high doses it causes both β_1- and β_2-agonist effects (+ inotropic, + chronotropic, vasodilator) and α-agonist effects (eg vasoconstriction). The latter, whilst increasing blood pressure, may reduce cardiac output ($\uparrow$ afterload), cause peripheral gangrene as well as increasing myocardial oxygen consumption and being pro-arrhythmogenic.

217 (a) False
    (b) True
    (c) True
    (d) True
    (e) False

The management of sinus tachycardia is directed to the underlying cause (e.g. pain, anxiety, left ventricular failure, asthma, thyrotoxicosis) and iatrogenic factors. Of calcium antagonists, verapamil causes bradycardia, dihyropyridines can cause reflex tachycardia, and diltiazem seldom causes appreciable changes in heart rate.

218 Lignocaine:

  (a) Is a class 1b agent that blocks cardiac Na^+ channels, reducing the rate of rise of the cardiac action potential and increasing the effective refractory period

  (b) Is epileptogenic

  (c) Is a positive inotrope

  (d) Is usually administered as an intravenous bolus followed by infusion

  (e) Is the drug of first choice for supraventricular tachycardia

219 The following prolong the QT interval:

  (a) Quinidine

  (b) Disopyramide

  (c) Phenytoin

  (d) Amitriptyline

  (e) Magnesium

220 Amiodarone:

  (a) Is indicated in resistant atrial fibrillation or flutter

  (b) Is effective in preventing recurrent ventricular fibrillation

  (c) Is contraindicated in Wolff–Parkinson–White (WPW) syndrome

  (d) May be given intravenously via a central line

  (e) Prolongs the QT interval

221 The following adverse effects are associated with amiodarone:

  (a) Visual disturbances (e.g. colored halos)

  (b) Hyperthyroidism

  (c) Hypothyroidism

  (d) Pulmonary fibrosis

  (e) Photosensitivity

222 Amiodarone:

  (a) Is highly lipid soluble

  (b) Has an apparent volume of distribution of approximately 5000 litres

  (c) Is predominantly eliminated by the kidney

  (d) Accumulates in the heart

  (e) Has a half-life of 28–45 days

223 Sotalol:

  (a) Is effective in supraventricular and ventricular arrythmias

  (b) Is not effective when given by mouth

  (c) The dose should be reduced in renal impairment

  (d) May cause torsades de pointes

  (e) Is a less potent negative inotrope than amiodarone

218 (a) True
    (b) True
    (c) False
    (d) True
    (e) False

Lignocaine has a narrow therapeutic index but is the drug of choice for the treatment of ventricular tachycardia and fibrillation (post-DC cardioconversion).

219 (a) True
    (b) True
    (c) False
    (d) True
    (e) False

A prolonged QT interval predisposes to torsades de pointes, a form of ventricular tachycardia.

220 (a) True
    (b) True
    (c) False
    (d) True
    (e) True

Amiodarone, a class III agent, is highly effective in both supraventricular and ventricular arrythmias. It is not a negative inotrope in contrast to most antiarrythmic agents.

221 (a) True
    (b) True
    (c) True
    (d) True
    (e) True

Adverse effects are many and varied and are common when plasma amiodarone concentration exceeds 2.5 mg/litre. Most are reversible on stopping treatment, but this is not true of pulmonary fibrosis.

222 (a) True
    (b) True
    (c) False
    (d) True
    (e) True

Amiodarone is highly protein bound and is slowly excreted by the liver. Antiarrhythmic activity may persist for several months after stopping treatment.

223 (a) True
    (b) False
    (c) True
    (d) True
    (e) False

Sotalol is a β-adrenoreceptor antagonist (class II) with additional class III antiarrhythmic activity.

224 Intravenous verapamil:

(a) May terminate supraventricular tachycardia
(b) Must not be given to patients receiving β-blockers
(c) Reduces digoxin excretion
(d) One must delay DC cardioversion at least 2 hours after a dose
(e) Shortens the PR interval

225 Adenosine:

(a) Is used to terminate ventricular tachycardia
(b) Is contraindicated in regular broad complex tachycardia
(c) Dilates bronchial smooth muscle
(d) Is associated with chest pain
(e) Circulatory effects last 20–30 seconds

226 Digoxin:

(a) Reduces the ventricular rate in atrial fibrillation
(b) Is contraindicated in second degree heart block
(c) Is the treatment of choice in atrial fibrillation in a patient with WPW
(d) Induced arrhythmias may be terminated by magnesium
(e) 80% of administered digoxin is excreted unchanged in the bile

227 A 70-year-old woman has recurrent, symptomatic ventricular tachycardia following an acute myocardial infarction in spite of DC conversion and lignocaine. The following may be effective:

(a) Amiodarone
(b) Bretylium
(c) Verapamil
(d) Adenosine
(e) Isoprenaline

228 The following are indications for transvenous pacing:

(a) Symptomatic sinus bradycardia post-inferior myocardial infarction
(b) First degree heart block post-inferior myocardial infarction
(c) A heart rate of 34 bpm at rest in an athlete with second degree (Mobitz type I) heart block
(d) Asymptomatic congenital complete heart block
(e) Blackouts associated with bradycardia in sick sinus syndrome

229 The following arrhythmias are correctly paired with their first line treatment:

(a) Ventricular fibrillation – synchronized DC cardioversion
(b) Ventricular fibrillation – unsynchronized DC cardioversion
(c) Ventricular tachycardia – propranolol
(d) Rapid atrial fibrillation – flecainide
(e) Drug-induced torsades de pointes – Disopyramide

224 **(a) True**   Verapamil slows intracardiac conduction affecting in particular
    (b) True   the AV node but also the SA node. It is a potent negative
    (c) True   inotrope. It should be avoided in WPW as it can increase
    (d) False   conduction through an accessory pathway.
    (e) False

225 **(a) False**   Adenosine is used to terminate supraventricular tachycardia
    (b) False   (SVT). It is particularly useful diagnostically in patients with
    (c) False   regular broad complex tachycardia which is suspected of
    (d) True   being SVT with aberrant conduction. If adenosine terminates
    (e) True   the bradycardia the AV node is involved.

226 **(a) True**   The main use of digoxin as an antiarrhythmic is to control the
    (b) True   ventricular rate (and hence improve cardiac output) in patients
    (c) False   with atrial fibrillation. Drugs causing hypokalemia aggravate
    (d) True   digoxin toxicity.
    (e) False

227 **(a) True**   Isoprenaline, a β-agonist is likely to be arrhythmogenic and
    (b) True   will increase myocardial oxygen consumption. Verapamil is a
    (c) False   potent negative inotrope and is only effective in supra-
    (d) False   ventricular tachycardia.
    (e) False

228 **(a) False**   Bradycardia and first degree heart block are common post
    (b) False   inferior myocardial infarction. If the bradycardia causes
    (c) False   symptoms 0.6 mg atropine IV is usually effective.
    (d) False
    (e) True

229 **(a) False**   If causing immediate cardiovascular embarassment, DC
    (b) True   cardioversion is indicated in ventricular tachycardia. Other-
    (c) False   wise, if intravenous lignocaine is ineffective, or oral
    (d) False   prophylaxis is required, amiodarone may be used.
    (e) False

5 RESPIRATORY SYSTEM

230 The following should be administered in acute severe asthma in an otherwise well 17-year-old man:
   (a) Continuous high percentage oxygen
   (b) Nebulized salbutamol
   (c) Intravenous corticosteroids
   (d) Nebulized ipratropium
   (e) Intravenous chlorpromazine

231 β_2-Agonists (e.g. salbutamol, terbutaline):
   (a) Relax bronchial smooth muscle
   (b) Inhibit release of mast cell and other inflammatory mediators
   (c) Reduce heart rate
   (d) Cause vasoconstriction
   (e) Decrease intracellular cyclic adenosine monophosphate (cAMP)

232 Adverse effects of salmeterol include:
   (a) Tremor
   (b) Palpitations
   (c) Hyperkalemia
   (d) Interstitial nephritis
   (e) Seizures

233 Inhaled corticosteroids (e.g. beclomethasone) when used to treat asthma:
   (a) Are contraindicated in growing children
   (b) Should be administered immediately before a β_2-agonist
   (c) Maximum alleviation of symptoms usually occurs within 24 hours of starting inhaled corticosteroid
   (d) Should not be prescribed if there is evidence of a respiratory tract infection
   (e) Cause hyperkalemia

234 Ipratropium bromide:
   (a) Is administered intravenously
   (b) Has an antimuscarinic action
   (c) Has no place in maintenance therapy of asthma
   (d) Has a bitter taste
   (e) Cannot be administered concurrently with β_2-agonists

235 Theophylline:
   (a) Is usually administered via an inhaler
   (b) Inhibits phosphodiesterase
   (c) Raises intracellular cAMP
   (d) Antagonizes adenosine at A_2-receptors
   (e) Is a metabolite of caffeine

230 **(a)** True   Intravenous fluids are administered to correct/prevent
    (b) True   dehydration. Antibiotics are administered if there is history/
    (c) True   signs of infection. Refractory cases require intravenous
    (d) True β_2-agonist (salbutamol) or theophylline. If these are inade-
    (e) False   quate, intermittent positive pressure ventilation is required.

231 **(a)** True β_2-Agonists stimulate adenylyl cyclase and increase intra-
    (b) True   cellular cAMP.
    (c) False
    (d) False
    (e) False

232 **(a)** True β_2-Agonists are generally well tolerated when given by
    (b) True   inhalation. Salmeterol, a long-acting β_2-agonist, is inhaled
    (c) False   twice daily.
    (d) False
    (e) False

233 **(a)** False   It is currently recommended that inhaled corticosteroids are
    (b) False   started when one inhaled dose of an inhaled β_2-agonist daily
    (c) False   fails to control symptoms.
    (d) False
    (e) False

234 **(a)** False   Inhaled antimuscarinic drugs such as ipratropium and
    (b) True   oxitropium are effective as acute and maintenance therapy in
    (c) False   asthma. High doses usually via a nebulizer may precipitate
    (d) True   acute glaucoma or urinary retention.
    (e) False

235 **(a)** False   Theophylline is adminstered via the oral route (usually in slow
    (b) True   release formulations) or the intravenous route (as the soluble
    (c) True   aminophylline) or rarely, via the rectal route.
    (d) True
    (e) False

236 Adverse effects associated with the use of theophylline include:

(a) Cardiac arrhythmias
(b) Convulsions
(c) Oral candidosis
(d) Sedation
(e) Nausea and vomiting

237 The following decrease the clearance of theophylline:

(a) Congestive cardiac failure
(b) CIrrhosis
(c) HIgh protein, low carbohydrate diet
(d) Concurrent ranitidine therapy
(e) Concurrent corticosteroid therapy

238 In acute severe asthma hydrocortisone:

(a) Is usually given via the intravenous route
(b) Subjective improvement takes 30–60 minutes
(c) Is contraindicated in growing children
(d) Is contraindicated in pregnancy
(e) Should be delayed until two doses of nebulized salbutamol have been administered

239 Administration of beclomethasone via an inhaler:

(a) Allows reduction in the maintenance dose of oral prednisolone in chronic asthma
(b) More of the dose is swallowed than enters the lungs
(c) Should be administered four times daily
(d) Has a lower systemic oral bioavailability than fluticasone
(e) Reversible inhibition of long bone growth occurs in children at high doses

240 Inhaled sodium cromoglycate:

(a) Is effective in alleviating an acute episode of allergic asthma
(b) Has no benefit in preventing exercise induced bronchospasm
(c) Prevents antigen–antibody combination
(d) Inhibits mediator release from mast cells
(e) May cause cardiac arrhythmias

236 **(a) True**   Theophylline has a narrow therapeutic index and the
     (b) True   pharmacokinetics show considerable interindividual variation.
     (c) False
     (d) False
     (e) True

237 **(a) True**   See Table 2 below.
     (b) True
     (c) False
     (d) False
     (e) False

Table 2   Factors influencing theophylline clearance.

Factors decreasing theophylline clearance and suggested dose (assuming normal dose is 100%)	Factors increasing theophyline clearance and suggested dose (assuming normal dose is 100%)
Congestive cardiac failure (40%)	Smoking (150%)
Hepatic disease cirrhosis (40%)	Marijuana (150%)
Old age (80%)	Barbecued meat (130%)
Neonates (60%)	Hyperthyroidism (150%)
Pneumonia (70%)	Drugs
Drugs	Carbamazepine (150%)
Cimetidine (50%)	Phenytoin (150%)
Erythromycin (75%)	Rifampicin (150%)
Chloramphenicol (75%)	Ethanol (120%)
Propranolol (70%)	High protein, low carbohydrate diet
Ciprofloxacin (50%)	(150%)
Interferon (75%)	

238 **(a) True**   Objective improvement does not occur until 6 hours and is
     (b) False   maximal 13 hours after the start of intravenous corticosteroid
     (c) False   treatment in asthma. This delay is due to the
     (d) False   pharmacodynamics of glucocorticoids which work via new
     (e) False   protein synthesis.

239 **(a) True**   Systemic adverse events are rarely significant with inhaled
     (b) True   glucocorticoids which are valuable in the prophylaxis of
     (c) False   asthma.
     (d) False
     (e) True

240 **(a) False**   Sodium cromoglycate is administered by inhalation of a
     (b) False   powder. Used prophylactically it can prevent type I and type III
     (c) False   allergic reactions and exercise provoked asthma. It is very
     (d) True   safe although approximately 1:10 000 experience broncho-
     (e) False   spasm or hoarseness.

241 The following antiasthma drugs are associated with hypokalemia:

    (a) Inhaled salbutamol
    (b) Intravenous theophylline
    (c) Oral prednisolone
    (d) Subcutaneous terbutaline
    (e) Inhaled sodium cromoglycate

242 The following drugs can produce pulmonary fibrosis:

    (a) Aspirin
    (b) Cyclophosphamide
    (c) Busulphan
    (d) Captopril
    (e) Amiodarone

241 (a) **True**   In acute severe asthma the electrolytes must be monitored.
    (b) **True**
    (c) **True**
    (d) **True**
    (e) **False**

242 (a) **False**   Captopril is associated with a dose-dependent chronic dry
    (b) **True**   cough. Aspirin (and nitrofurantoin, imipramine, isoniazid,
    (c) **True**   penicillins and streptomycin) has been associated with
    (d) **False**   pulmonary eosinophilia.
    (e) **True**

6 ALIMENTARY SYSTEM

243 The following stimulate gastric acid secretion:

(a) Vagal stimulation
(b) Gastrin
(c) Acetylcholine stimulation of the M_1-receptor
(d) Histamine stimulation of the H_2-receptor
(e) Increased intracellular cAMP

244 Prostaglandin E_2:

(a) Is the principal prostaglandin synthesized in the stomach
(b) Stimulates gastric acid secretion
(c) Causes vasoconstriction of submucosal blood vessels
(d) Biosynthesis is inhibited by aspirin
(e) Biosynthesis is inhibited by rectal indomethacin

243 **(a) True**
   (b) True
   (c) True
   (d) True
   (e) True

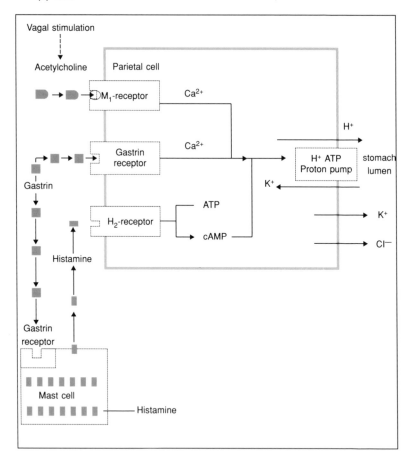

Fig. 2 Mechanisms regulating hydrochloric acid secretion. Ca^{2+}, calcium; ATP, adenosine triphosphate; cAMP, cyclic adenosine monophosphate; K^+, potassium; Cl^-, chloride

244 **(a) True**   Prostaglandin E_2 is an important gastroprotective mediator. It
   (b) False   inhibits secretion of acid, promotes secretion of protective
   (c) False   mucus and causes vasodilation of submucosal blood vessels.
   (d) True
   (e) True

245 *Helicobacter pylori:*

    (a) Is strongly linked to the development of carcinoma of the colon

    (b) Is a bacterium that is strongly linked to the development and recurrence of duodenal ulcer

    (c) Is usually found in the gastric antrum

    (d) Is uncommon in asymptomatic patients

    (e) Colonization of the stomach is inhibited by corticosteroids

246 The following accelerate healing in gastric ulcers:

    (a) Bed rest

    (b) Stopping smoking

    (c) Corticosteroids

    (d) Cimetidine

    (e) Sucralfate

247 Antacids:

    (a) Large doses heal gastric ulcers more frequently than duodenal ulcers

    (b) Standard doses reduce gastric acidity for approximately 4 hours

    (c) Magnesium salts tend to cause diarrhea

    (d) Aluminum salts tend to cause a diuresis

    (e) Magnesium and aluminum salts reduce the rate and extent of absorption of phenytoin

248 Cimetidine therapy is associated with:

    (a) Transient increase in serum prolactin

    (b) Irreversible gynecomastia

    (c) Mental confusion in the elderly

    (d) Asystole after rapid intravenous injection

    (e) Reversible rise in serum creatinine

249 Cimetidine reduces the absorption of:

    (a) Ketoconazole

    (b) Pancreatic enzymes administered in pancreatic insufficiency

    (c) Penicillin V

    (d) Salicylate

    (e) Ferrous sulfate

250 In comparison to cimetidine, ranitidine:

    (a) Does not bind to androgen receptors

    (b) Is less likely to cause gynecomastia

    (c) Penetrates the blood brain barrier to a lesser extent

    (d) Is not available for parenteral use

    (e) Has a lower affinity for cytochrome P_{450}

245 **(a) False**   *Helicobacter pylori* is strongly linked to the development and
    (b) True   recurrence of duodenal ulcer. Possible linkage to gastric
    (c) True   carcinoma is under investigation.
    (d) False
    (e) False

246 **(a) True** – But unnecessary due to efficacy of current treatment
    (b) True – More effective in preventing recurrence of duodenal ulcers than
            H_2-blockers
    (c) False – Ulcerogenic
    (d) True
    (e) True

247 **(a) False**   Antacids produce prompt but transient pain relief in patients
    (b False   with peptic ulceration. Aluminum salts cause constipation.
    (c) True
    (d) False
    (e) True

248 **(a) True**   Chronic cimetidine therapy causes reversible gynecomastia in
    (b) False   0.1–0.2% of patients. It is generally well tolerated.
    (c) True
    (d) True
    (e) True

249 **(a) True**   Cimetidine reduces the absorption of drugs which require a
    (b) False   low pH. It improves the efficacy of oral pancreatic enzymes
    (c) False   which are inactivated by gastric acid.
    (d) False
    (e) False

250 **(a) True**   All the H_2-receptor blockers currently available in the UK are
    (b) True   effective in peptic ulceration and are well tolerated. There is
    (c) True   most experience with cimetidine and ranitidine.
    (d) False
    (e) True

251 Omeprazole:

    (a) Is an irreversible inhibitor of the hydrogen/potassium adenosine triphosphatase locus of the gastric parietal cell

    (b) Reduces gastric acid secretion

    (c) Is the drug of choice in Zollinger–Ellison syndrome

    (d) Has a plasma half-life of approximately 1 hour

    (e) Requires dose reduction in renal failure

252 Omeprazole enhances the effects of the following drugs through inhibition of drug metabolism:

    (a) Atenolol

    (b) Amoxycillin

    (c) Captopril

    (d) Warfarin

    (e) Phenytoin

253 Misoprostol:

    (a) Is a synthetic analog of prostaglandin E

    (b) Inhibits cyclo-oxygenase

    (c) Causes vasodilatation in the submucosa

    (d) Is rapidly and nearly completely absorbed

    (e) Is contraindicated in pregnancy

254 Pirenzepine, a muscarinic receptor antagonist:

    (a) Is a selective M_1-receptor antagonist

    (b) Decreases gastric acid secretion

    (c) Increases gastric motility

    (d) Causes decreased salivation

    (e) Is contraindicated in narrow angle glaucoma

255 Bismuth chelate

    (a) Precipitates at acid pH

    (b) Stimulates mucus production

    (c) Has a direct toxic effect on *Heliobacter pylori*

    (d) Causes pale stools

    (e) Causes nausea

256 Sucralfate

    (a) Requires systemic absorption for anti-ulcer activity

    (b) Contains aluminum

    (c) Is effective in healing gastric ulcers

    (d) Is contraindicated in pregnancy

    (e) Is associated with constipation

251 (a) **True**　Omeprazole, a proton pump inhibitor, is most effective in
　　(b) **True**　reducing gastric secretion and in spite of its short half-life only
　　(c) **True**　has to be administered once daily since it acts irreversibly.
　　(d) **True**
　　(e) **False**

252 (a) **False**　For drugs such as phenytoin and warfarin which have a
　　(b) **False**　narrow therapeutic index this is clinically significant.
　　(c) **False**
　　(d) **True**
　　(e) **True**

253 (a) **True**　Misoprostol inhibits gastric acid secretion, causes vasodilata-
　　(b) **False**　tion in the submucosa and stimulates production of protective
　　(c) **True**　mucus. It contracts uterine muscle and causes abortion.
　　(d) **True**
　　(e) **True**

254 (a) **True**　Of the muscarinic receptor antagonists only pirenzepine has
　　(b) **True**　significant antisecretory effects at a tolerated dose.
　　(c) **False**
　　(d) **True**
　　(e) **True**

255 (a) **True**　Several studies show bismuth chelate to be as active as
　　(b) **True**　cimetidine in the healing of duodenal and gastric ulcers after
　　(c) **True**　4–8 weeks of treatment. It is, however, associated with
　　(d) **False**　frequent minor adverse effects. It is a part of "triple therapy"
　　(e) **True**　for the eradication of *H. pylori*.

256 (a) **False**　Sucralfate, a basic aluminum salt, becomes a sticky adherent
　　(b) **True**　paste in the presence of acid which retains antacid efficacy
　　(c) **True**　and apparently coats the floor of ulcer craters.
　　(d) **False**
　　(e) **True**

257 The following drugs are used to prevent motion sickness:

(a) Hyoscine
(b) Promethazine
(c) Cinnarizine
(d) Metoclopramide
(e) Chlorpromazine

258 Cyclizine:

(a) Is a dopamine receptor antagonist
(b) Is effective in morphine-induced vomiting
(c) Is a proven teratogen
(d) Causes dry mouth
(e) Causes drowsiness

259 Metoclopramide:

(a) Is most effective in centrally mediated vomiting
(b) Is ineffective in drug-induced nausea
(c) Increases the rate of gastric emptying
(d) Should be avoided for 3–4 days following gastrointestinal surgery
(e) High doses block $5HT_3$ receptors

260 Acute dystonic reactions related to metoclopramide:

(a) Occur in approximately 10% of patients
(b) Include trismus
(c) Are more common in males
(d) Can be treated with benztropine
(e) Can be treated with diazepam

261 Ondansetron:

(a) Is a phenothiazine
(b) Is not absorbed after oral administration
(c) Is effective in preventing nausea and vomiting due to cancer
    chemotherapy and radiotherapy
(d) Is ineffective in ciplastin induced nausea
(e) 1% of patients have dystonic reactions

262 In ulcerative colitis:

(a) Intravenous hydrocortisone is of proven value in the treatment of acute
    colitis
(b) Oral corticosteroids are first line for maintenance treatment
(c) Localized rectal disease often responds to prednisolone enemas/
    suppositories
(d) In severe colitis codeine should be used
(e) Fiber is contraindicated

257 **(a) True** – Muscarinic antagonist; NB: anticholinergic side effects
   (b) True – H_1-blocker minor anti-muscarinic action
   (c) True – H_1-blocker minor anti-muscarinic action
   (d) False – Dopamine receptor antagonist
   (e) False – Chlorpromazine is not used for motion sickness

258 **(a) False** – H_1-blocker with additional antimuscarinic actions
   (b) True
   (c) False
   (d) True
   (e) True

259 **(a) False** – Relatively ineffective in motion sickness and other forms of centrally mediated vomiting
   (b) False
   (c) True – Increases the rate of absorption of oral drugs
   (d) True
   (e) True – Effective in some patients in preventing cisplatin-induced nausea and vomiting

260 **(a) False** – About 1%
   (b) True – Also akathisia, oculogyric crises, torticollis and opisthotonos
   (c) False – Commoner in females and the young
   (d) True
   (e) True

261 **(a) False** – Ondansetron is a highly selective $5HT_3$-receptor antagonist
   (b) False – Is used both orally and intravenously
   (c) True
   (d) False
   (e) False – Occasionally causes constipation

262 **(a) True** – Correction of dehydration, nutritional and electrolyte imbalance are life-saving
   (b) False – Because of side effects
   (c) True – Some systemic absorption may occur
   (d) False – May precipitate paralytic ileus and megacolon
   (e) False – A high fiber diet and bulk-forming drugs are useful in adjusting fecal consistency

263 Sulfasalazine:

    (a) Is a prodrug
    (b) Is used for maintenance treatment of ulcerative colitis
    (c) Is not effective in small bowel Crohn's disease
    (d) May be administered orally or rectally
    (e) Should be avoided in G6PD deficiency

264 Adverse effects associated with sulfasalazine include:

    (a) Blood dyscrasias
    (b) Oligospermia
    (c) Stevens–Johnson syndrome
    (d) SLE-like syndrome
    (e) Hepatitis

265 Mesalazine:

    (a) Is a prodrug consisting of a dimer of two 5-aminosalicylic acid molecules
    (b) Dissolves at the pH found in the terminal ileum and colon
    (c) Is contraindicated in sulfonamide hypersensitivity
    (d) Is associated with oligospermia
    (e) Is associated with interstitial nephritis

266 The following drugs cause constipation:

    (a) Amiodarone
    (b) Amitriptyline
    (c) Amoxycillin
    (d) Misoprostol
    (e) Metformin

267 Lactulose:

    (a) Is a chemical stimulant to the colon
    (b) Produces its effect 10–12 hours after an oral dose
    (c) Requires colonic bacteria for activity
    (d) Should not be administered concurrently with bran
    (e) Is contraindicated in liver failure

268 Loperamide:

    (a) Decreases intestinal transit time
    (b) Increases bulk of gut contents
    (c) Requires systemic absorption for activity on the bowel
    (d) Causes pupil constriction
    (e) Causes hypersalivation

263 **(a) True**   – Broken down to 5-aminosalicylate and sulfapyridine
    (b) True
    (c) True
    (d) True
    (e) True

264 **(a) True**   Adverse effects are more common in slow acelylators.
    (b) True
    (c) True
    (d) True
    (e) True

265 **(a) False** – This describes olsalazine
    (b) True
    (c) False – But is contraindicated in salicylate hypersensitivity
    (d) False
    (e) True   – Contraindicated in renal impairment

266 **(a) True**   The cause of any change in bowel habit should be deter-
    (b) True   mined before laxatives are used.
    (c) False
    (d) False
    (e) False

267 **(a) False**   Lactulose is a disaccharide which is broken down in the colon
    (b) False   by bacteria to unabsorbed organic anions which retain fluid in
    (c) True   the gut lumen.
    (d) False
    (e) False

268 **(a) False** – Loperamide increases intestinal transit time
    (b) False   See *CPT*, Chapter 31, p. 416.
    (c) False
    (d) False
    (e) False

269 Treatment of hepatic encephalopathy includes:

  (a) Dietary protein restriction
  (b) Emptying the lower bowel
  (c) Oral lactulose
  (d) Chlorpheniramine
  (e) Oral methionine

270 The emergency drug therapy of portal hypertension and esophageal varices may include:

  (a) Vasopressin
  (b) Chenodeoxycholic acid
  (c) Calcitonin
  (d) Octreotide
  (e) Isoprenaline

271 The following drugs are associated with cholestatic jaundice/hepatitis:

  (a) HMGCoA reductase inhibitors
  (b) Methotrexate
  (c) Synthetic estrogens
  (d) Chlorpromazine
  (e) Rifampicin

272 The long-term efficacy and safety of the following drugs in reducing obesity has been established:

  (a) Thyroxine
  (b) Diethylpropion
  (c) Thiazide diuretics
  (d) Pizotifen
  (e) Mazindol

269 **(a) True**   See _CPT_, Chapter 31, p. 418–9.
    (b) True
    (c) True
    (d) False
    (e) False

270 **(a) True**   See _CPT_, Chapter 31, p. 419.
    (b) False
    (c) False
    (d) True
    (e) False

271 **(a) False** – Usually mild and asymptomatic increase in transaminases
    (b) False – Hepatic fibrosis/cirrhosis
    (c) True – Rare now low dose estrogens are more commonly prescribed
    (d) True – Estimated incidence 0.5% associated with fever, abdominal pain
                    and pruritus
    (e) True – Usually transient

272 **(a) False** – Dangerous and irrational in euthyroid patients
    (b) False – Related to amphetamine – abuse potential
    (c) False – Transient weight loss secondary to fluid loss
    (d) False – Inhibits $5HT_2$-receptors, increases appetite and causes weight
                    gain
    (e) False – Long-term efficacy not established

7 ENDOCRINE SYSTEM

273 In young insulin-dependent diabetic (IDDM) patients:

   (a) There is good evidence that improved diabetic control reduces the incidence of microvascular complications
   (b) Blood glucose monitoring should be performed at home
   (c) Once-daily subcutaneous insulin usually provides acceptable control
   (d) The carbohydrate content should be 45–55% of total calories
   (e) A fiber-rich diet reduces peak plasma glucose after meals and reduces insulin requirements

274 Recombinant human insulin in diabetes mellitus:

   (a) Never produces allergic reactions
   (b) The effective dose may be less than animal insulin
   (c) Patients are less aware of hypoglycemia
   (d) Should not be given intravenously
   (e) Is not available as a long-acting preparation

275 A 17-year-old woman is admitted comatose with diabetic ketoacidosis. The following is accepted practice:

   (a) 500 ml of 0.9% saline in the first two hours
   (b) Bladder catheterization
   (c) Subcutaneous insulin 0.1 unit/kg/hour
   (d) 8.4% intravenous bicarbonate if the arterial pH is betwen 7.2 and 7.3
   (e) Aspiration of the stomach

276 Sulfonylureas:

   (a) Are used in obese diabetics who show a tendency to ketosis
   (b) Improve symptoms of polyuria and polydipsia
   (c) Have been shown to reduce the vascular complications of non-insulin dependent diabetes mellitus (NIDDM)
   (d) Require functioning β-cells for a hypoglycemic effect
   (e) Are usually administered once daily at bed time

277 Gliclazide:

   (a) Is a sulfonylurea
   (b) Has a shorter half-life than chlorpropamide
   (c) Hypoglycemia can be reversed by intramuscular glucagon
   (d) Should not be prescribed concurrently with metformin
   (e) Stimulates appetite

278 Metformin, a biguanide:

   (a) May cause lactic acidosis
   (b) Is particularly useful in alcoholic diabetic patients
   (c) Causes hypoglycemia in non-diabetic patients
   (d) Should be discontinued before major elective surgery
   (e) Causes anorexia and weight loss

273 **(a) True**   In IDDM, in addition to tight diabetic control which can usually
    (b) True   be achieved by education and insulin three times daily plus
    (c) False   diet, there must be regular screening for microvascular
    (d) True   complications. Laser therapy of early proliferative retinopathy
    (e) True   prevents blindness.

274 **(a) False** – But less common than with animal insulin
    (b) True – Possibly due to fewer blocking antibodies
    (c) False – Initial fears unfounded following double blind studies
    (d) False
    (e) False

275 **(a) False** – 1.5–2 litres over the first 2 hours
    (b) True – Helps in accurate monitoring of urine output. A central venous
                 pressure line also aids fluid management
    (c) False – Give intravenous insulin via syringe pump
    (d) False – May worsen intracellular and cerebrospinal acidemia
    (e) True – Gastric stasis is common and inhalation of vomit can be fatal.
                  Insertion of a cuffed endotracheal tube may be necessary before
                  nasogastric aspiration

276 **(a) False**
    (b) True
    (c) False
    (d) True – Increase plasma insulin levels
    (e) False – Most commonly as a single dose with breakfast

277 **(a) True**
    (b) True
    (c) True – A useful alternative to intravenous glucose if venous access is
                  impractical (e.g. in the home)
    (d) False
    (e) True – cf. metformin

278 **(a) True**   Metformin is useful in obese patients with NIDDM uncontrolled
    (b) False   by diet and a sulfonylurea. The anorexia is useful in obese
    (c) False   diabetic patients. Lactic acidosis is the most sinister adverse
    (d) True   effect and has a mortality of approximately 60%. It is contra-
    (e) True   indicated in renal/hepatic/cardiac failure.

279 Carbimazole:

    (a) Decreases thyroid hormone synthesis
    (b) Inhibits the peripheral conversion of T4 to the more active T3
    (c) Is safe in pregnancy
    (d) Has an active metabolite
    (e) Is associated with neutropenia

280 The following may cause hypercalcemia:

    (a) Plicamycin
    (b) Calcitonin
    (c) Bisphosphonates
    (d) Excess vitamin D
    (e) Thiazide diuretics

281 Disodium etidronate is used:

    (a) By intramuscular injection
    (b) In Paget's disease
    (c) In hypercalcemia of malignancy
    (d) With calcium carbonate in established vertebral osteoporosis
    (e) To inhibit bone resorption and formation

282 Glucocorticoids:

    (a) Reduce circulating numbers of eosinophils
    (b) Reduce circulating numbers of T lymphocytes
    (c) Increase circulating numbers of neutrophils
    (d) Increase circulating numbers of platelets
    (e) Inhibit the production of lipocortin

283 Rapid withdrawal after prolonged prednisolone administration can cause:

    (a) Acute adrenal insufficiency
    (b) Malaise
    (c) Fever
    (d) Arthralgia
    (e) Raised intracranial pressure

284 Chronic administration of corticosteroids (iatrogenic Cushing's syndrome) results in:

    (a) Increased susceptibility to opportunistic infection
    (b) Hyperkalemia
    (c) Hypertension
    (d) Posterior capsular cataracts
    (e) Proximal myopathy

279 (a) True
    (b) False – Cf. propylthiouracil and β-blockers
    (c) False
    (d) True – Methimazole, which is responsible for the therapeutic action
    (e) True – Potentially fatal

280 (a) False   Hypercalcemia may be a life-threatening emergency. General
    (b) False   management includes maintenance of hydration with physio-
    (c) False   logical saline. Plicamycin, calcitonin and bisphosphonates
    (d) True   reduce the plasma calcium. Glucocoritcoids reduce plasma
    (e) True   calcium in sarcoidosis.

281 (a) False   Is given intravenously or orally in spite of poor systemic
    (b) True   availability (1–5%). It is generally well tolerated.
    (c) True
    (d) True
    (e) True

282 (a) True   Glucocorticoids induce the synthesis of lipocortin which
    (b) True   inhibits phospholipase A_2 and consequently inhibits the
    (c) True   formation of several pro-inflammatory mediators.
    (d) True
    (e) False

283 (a) True   Even in patients who have been successfully weaned from
    (b) True   chronic steroid therapy, an acute stress (e.g. trauma, surgery,
    (c) True   infection) may precipitate an acute adrenal crisis.
    (d) True
    (e) True

284 (a) True – (e.g. fungi and TB – may reactivate old tuberculous lesions)
    (b) False – Hypokalemia
    (c) True
    (d) True – + local application of steroids to the eye encourages infection
    (e) True

285 Oral prednisolone therapy is indicated in:

   (a) Fibrosing alveolitis
   (b) Temporal arteritis
   (c) Peptic ulceration
   (d) Diabetes mellitus
   (e) Idiopathic thrombocytopenic purpura

286 The risk of thromboembolic disease associated with the combined oral contraceptive is increased in women:

   (a) Over 35 years of age
   (b) Who smoke
   (c) Who have been using oral contraceptives for 5 years or more continuously
   (d) Who use inhaled beclomethasone for asthma
   (e) Who have a history of thromboembolism

287 Adverse effects associated with the combined oral contraceptive include:

   (a) Aggravation of asthma
   (b) Stroke in women with migraine
   (c) Nephrotic syndrome
   (d) Peripheral neuropathy
   (e) Budd–Chiari syndrome

288 Bromocriptine

   (a) Stimulates lactation
   (b) Is used to treat hyperprolactinemia
   (c) Is a dopamine D_2-receptor agonist
   (d) Commonly causes diarrhea
   (e) Is effective in reducing symptoms of carcinoid syndrome

285 **(a) True**   – Not curative but delays deterioriation in some patients
    (b) True   – May save sight
    (c) False
    (d) False
    (e) True

286 **(a) True**   The combined oral contraceptive should be stopped 4 weeks
    (b) True   before major elective surgery.
    (c) True
    (d) False
    (e) True

287 **(a) False**   The overall acceptability of the combined pill is 80%: minor
    (b) True   side effects can often be controlled by a change in
    (c) False   preparation.
    (d) False
    (e) True

288 **(a) False** – Suppresses lactation
    (b) True
    (c) True
    (d) False – The commonest adverse effects are nausea and constipation
    (e) False – Octreotide, a synthetic analog of somatostatin is used

8 SELECTIVE TOXICITY

289 The following drugs are bacteriostatic rather than bactericidal at doses normally used in clinical practice:

(a) Penicillins
(b) Aminoglycosides
(c) Erythromycin
(d) Tetracycline
(e) Ciprofloxacin

290 The following antibacterial drugs inhibit folic acid metabolism:

(a) Penicillins
(b) Monobactams
(c) Quinolones
(d) Trimethoprim
(e) Sulfonamides

291 The following infections have been paired with appropriate antibacterial therapy:

(a) Acute otitis media – amoxycillin
(b) Acute epiglottitis in children – chloramphenicol or cefotaxime
(c) Legionnaire's disease – erythromycin and rifampicin
(d) Acute cystitis arising outside hospital in adults – trimethoprim
(e) Antibiotic-associated pseudomembranous colitis – oral vancomycin

292 The following antibacterial drug combinations are of accepted benefit in the treatment of the infection cited:

(a) Amoxycillin and cephadroxil for lower urinary tract infection in severely ill patients
(b) Phenoxymethylpenicillin and tetracycline for acute osteomyelitis in a child under 5 years
(c) Isoniazid, rifampicin and pyrazinamide for pulmonary TB
(d) Erythromycin and tetracycline for septicemia
(e) Metronidazole and nitrofurantoin for non-specific urethritis

293 The following antibacterial drugs are suitable as prophylaxis in the conditions cited:

(a) Co-amoxiclav – human and animal bites
(b) Clprofloxacin – close adult contacts of meningoccal disease
(c) Flucloxacillin – prevention of a secondary case of diphtheria
(d) Erythromycin – whooping cough contact in an unvaccinated child under 1 year old
(e) Penicillin – traumatic CSF leakage (e.g. skull base fracture)

289 (a) **False**   In clinical practice the distinction is seldom important unless
    (b) **False**   the body's defense mechanisms are depressed.
    (c) **True**
    (d) **True**
    (e) **False**

290 (a) **False** – Inhibit cell wall synthesis
    (b) **False** – Inhibit cell wall synthesis
    (c) **False** – Inhibit DNA gyrase
    (d) **True**
    (e) **True**

291 (a) **True** – When bacterial commonly caused by group A streptococci
    (b) **True** – Caused by *H. influenzae*
    (c) **True**
    (d) **True**
    (e) **True** – Alternative oral metronidazole (NB: stop causative antibiotic)

292 (a) **False** – Intravenous gentamicin and cefuroxime
    (b) **False** – May be *Haemophilus influenzae* or *Staph. aureus* – amoxycillin
              and flucloxacillin is usually a satisfactory combination
    (c) **True** – Reduces the risk of resistance
    (d) **False** – Choice depends on clinical conditions, a penicillin and an
              aminoglycoside are a common combination in septicemia
    (e) **False** – Single agent effective (e.g. tetracycline or erythromycin)

293 (a) **True**
    (b) **True**
    (c) **False** – Erythromycin
    (d) **True**
    (e) **True**

294 Benzylpenicillin:

(a) Is inactivated in gastric acid
(b) Is effective in streptococcal, pneumococcal and meningococcal infections
(c) Has a half-life of approximately 12 hours
(d) Is less susceptible than flucloxacillin to β-lactamase-producing strains of staphylococci
(e) Approximately 1 in 500 injections cause anaphylaxis

295 Amoxycillin:

(a) Unlike benzylpenicillin is not susceptible to β-lactamases
(b) Is effective against many strains of H. influenzae
(c) Is ineffective in most urinary tract infections
(d) Drug-related skin rashes may appear after dosing has stopped
(e) Drug-related skin rashes are more common in a patients with infectious mononucleosis

296 The following drugs are commonly effective in staphylococcal infections:

(a) Ampicillin
(b) Co-amoxiclav
(c) Fusidic acid
(d) Flucloxacillin
(e) Metronidazole

297 Cefuroxime:

(a) Has activity against streptococci
(b) Has no activity against Gram-negative organisms
(c) Plasma concentrations should be monitored to avoid toxicity
(d) Is principally renally eliminated
(e) Has 10% cross-sensitivity for allergic reactions with benzylpenicillin

298 Gentamicin, an aminoglycoside:

(a) Is effective in pneumococcal pneumonia
(b) Is poorly absorbed from the gut
(c) Has an elimination half-life of approximately 12 hours if renal function is normal
(d) Cerebrospinal fluid (CSF) penetration is poor
(e) Causes irreversible eighth nerve damage

299 Chloramphenicol is usually effective in:

(a) Pulmonary tuberculosis
(b) Epiglottitis
(c) Typhoid
(d) Bacterial meningitis
(e) Bacterial conjunctivitis

294 **(a) True**
  (b) True
  (c) False – Short half-life of approximately 30 minutes
  (d) False
  (e) False – 1 in 100 000

295 **(a) False**   Amoxycillin is an extended-range penicillin used for a variety
  (b) True   of chest infections, otitis media, urinary tract infection, biliary
  (c) False   infections and prevention of bacterial endocarditis. Rashes are
  (d) True   common and there is an especially high incidence in
  (e) True   infectious mononucleosis and lymphatic leukemia.

296 **(a) False** – Susceptible to β-lactamases
  (b) True – A combination of amoxycillin with clavulanic acid (a β-lactamase
            inhibitor)
  (c) True
  (d) True
  (e) False

297 **(a) True**   Cefuroxime combines lactamase stability with activity against
  (b) False   streptococci, staphylococci, *H. influenzae* and *E. coli*.
  (c) False
  (d) True
  (e) True

298 **(a) False**   Aminoglycosides are used particularly in serious infections
  (b) True   such as septicemia usually in combination with a penicillin.
  (c) False   Blood concentration monitoring is mandatory to avoid toxicity.
  (d) True   The half-life is approximately 2 hours if renal function is
  (e) True   normal.

299 **(a) False**   Chloramphenicol has a broad spectrum and penetrates
  (b) True   tissues exceptionally well. Its widespread use in developing
  (c) True   countries has led to some resistance. Its major disadvantage
  (d) True   is a 1:40 000 incidence of aplastic anemia.
  (e) True

300 Uses of erythromycin include:

   (a) *Mycoplasma pneumoniae*
   (b) Legionnaire's disease
   (c) *Campylobacter enteritis*
   (d) Non-specific urethritis
   (e) Meningococcal meningitis

301 Erythromycin:

   (a) Is poorly absorbed when given by mouth
   (b) Has a shorter half-life (t½) than azithromycin
   (c) The most common adverse effect is headache
   (d) Inhibits cytochrome P_{450}
   (e) Cannot be prescribed with amoxycillin

302 Tetracyclines are used to treat:

   (a) Infections caused by *Clostridium difficile*
   (b) Lyme disease
   (c) Acne vulgaris
   (d) Systemic lupus erythematosus
   (e) Non-specific urethritis

303 Metronidazole is used to treat:

   (a) Trichomonal infections
   (b) Amebic dysentry
   (c) Giardiasis
   (d) Tetanus
   (e) Gas gangrene

304 Trimethoprim is:

   (a) Usually preferred to co-trimoxazole for the treatment of urinary tract infection
   (b) Generally preferred to co-trimoxazole for the treatment of pneumocystis pneumonia
   (c) Should be avoided in epileptic patients
   (d) Is effective treatment for Legionnaire's disease
   (e) Inhibits aldehyde dehydrogenase causing a disulfiram-like reaction with alcohol

305 Ciprofloxacin:

   (a) Is a drug of first choice effective in *Strep. pneumonae* infections
   (b) Is effective in *Pseudomonas* infections
   (c) Should be avoided in children
   (d) Should be avoided in epileptics
   (e) Is ineffective if administered orally

300 **(a) True**   Erythromycin, a macrolide, is a useful alternative to
    (b) True   penicillin in penicillin-allergic patients (with the notable
    (c) True   exception of meningitis) and is also effective against several
    (d) True   unusual bacteria.
    (e) False

301 **(a) False** – Well absorbed
    (b) True – Erythromycin $t_{\frac{1}{2}}$ 1–1.5 hours, azithromycin 40–60 hours
    (c) False – Gastro-intestinal effects are most common
    (d) True – Causes accumulation of theophylline, warfarin and terfenadine
    (e) False – Often co-prescribed in community acquired pneumonia

302 **(a) False**   Oral absorption of tetracyclines is reduced by food (except
    (b) True   doxycycline). They must be avoided in renal impairment
    (c) True   (except doxycycline).
    (d) False
    (e) True

303 **(a) True**   Metronidazole has high activity against amebae. It is widely
    (b) True   used prophylactically before abdominal surgery when the
    (c) True   rectal route is often suitable.
    (d) False
    (e) True

304 **(a) True**   Trimethoprim is generally preferred to co-trimoxazole
    (b) False   (trimethoprim + sulfamethoxazole) in all indications except
    (c) False   pneumocystis pneumonia. Hypersensitivity reactions including
    (d) False   Stevens–Johnson syndrome are relatively common with
    (e) False   sulfonamides.

305 **(a) False**   Oral bioavailability of the 4-fluoroquinolones is good and they
    (b) True   offer an oral alternative to parenteral aminoglycocides and
    (c) True   anti-pseudomonal penicillins for the treatment of pseudomonal
    (d) True   infection. Quinolones cause arthropathy in young animals and
    (e) False   can cause convulsions. Photosensitivity also occurs.

306 Isoniazid:

   (a) Is acetylated in the liver
   (b) Is used for only the initial 2 months of the recommended 6 month anti-TB regimen in the UK
   (c) Is readily absorbed from the gut
   (d) Does not diffuse into the CSF
   (e) Is contraindicated in children under the age of 10 years

307 Adverse effects associated with rifampicin include:

   (a) Hepatitis and cholestatic jaundice
   (b) Peripheral neuropathy
   (c) Convulsions
   (d) Influenza-like symptoms
   (e) Pink/red urine and tears

308 Rifampicin accelerates the metabolism of:

   (a) Corticosteroids
   (b) Warfarin
   (c) Streptomycin
   (d) Digoxin
   (e) Estrogen

309 The following adverse effects are correctly paired with a causative anti-tuberculous drug:

   (a) Peripheral neuropathy − isoniazid
   (b) Ototoxicity − rifampicin
   (c) Hyperuricemia − pyrazinamide
   (d) Retrobulbar neuritis − ethambutol
   (e) Hepatotoxicity − streptomycin

310 Dapsone:

   (a) Is used in the treatment of amebiasis
   (b) Is indicated in multibacillary leprosy
   (c) Is used in the treatment of dermatitis herpetiformis
   (d) Is acetylated in the liver
   (e) Has cross-sensitivity with sulfonamides

311 Amphotericin B:

   (a) Is effective in local *Candida* spp. infections
   (b) Is effective in systemic *Candida* spp. infections
   (c) Is nephrotoxic
   (d) Causes hypokalemia
   (e) Is ineffective in cryptococcosis

312 The following antifungal agents have been paired correctly with an appropriate indication:

- (a) Nystatin – oral *Candida* infections
- (b) Griseofulvin – cryptoccal pneumonia
- (c) Flucytosine – tinea pedis
- (d) Clotrimazole – intertrigo
- (e) Miconazole – cold sores

313 Ketoconazole:

- (a) Is effective as topical and oral therapy
- (b) Is active against *Aspergillus*
- (c) Inhibits cortisol biosynthesis
- (d) Blocks testosterone synthesis
- (e) Absorption is reduced by H_2-blockers

314 Fluconazole:

- (a) Oral absorption is minimal unless taken on an empty stomach
- (b) Presystemic metabolism is extensive
- (c) Penetrates the central nervous system well
- (d) Is excreted 80% by the kidney
- (e) Causes gynecomastia

315 Acyclovir:

- (a) Inhibits viral DNA synthesis
- (b) Is indicated in herpetic keratitis
- (c) Should be avoided if possible in pregnancy
- (d) Is indicated in herpetic meningoencephalitis
- (e) Is ineffective in chicken pox

316 Foscarnet:

- (a) Is indicated in cytomegalovirus (CMV) retinitis
- (b) Acyclovir-resistent herpes simplex virus infections
- (c) Is nephrotoxic
- (d) Causes fits
- (e) Is usually administered by mouth or topically

317 Adverse effects associated with the interferons include:

- (a) Hypocalcemia
- (b) Inhibition of spermatogenesis
- (c) Renal tubular acidosis
- (d) Lymphopenia
- (e) Influenza-like symptoms

318 One or more of the interferons are indicated in:

- (a) Herpes simplex encephalitis
- (b) Chronic hepatitis B infection
- (c) Chronic hepatitis C infection
- (d) Hairy cell leukemia
- (e) CMV retinitis

312 **(a) True** – NB: bitter taste
(b) False – Systemically active but limited to dermatophytes (ringworm fungi)
(c) False – Used with amphotericin for systemic candidosis and cryptococcosis
(d) True – Powder suitable
(e) False – Cold sores are due to herpes simplex

313 **(a) True**   The systemic use of ketoconazole has waned because of the
(b) False   high incidence of hepatic and endocrine side effects. It inhibits
(c) True   the metabolism of cyclosporin, terfenadine and astemizole.
(d) True
(e) True

314 **(a) False**   Fluconazole is potent and broad-spectrum antifungal drug.
(b) False   It may be used for local or systemic infections as well as
(c) True   prophylaxis in neutropenic patients. Adverse effects are
(d) True   gastrointestinal, erythema multiforme and hepatitis.
(e) False

315 **(a) True**   Acyclovir is a potent and selective inhibitor of herpes viruses.
(b) True   It may be administered as an ointment (e.g. in herpetic
(c) True   keratitis), orally (as in shingles) or by intravenous infusion as
(d) True   in encephalitis.
(e) False

316 **(a) True**   Foscarnet is a nucleotide analog that inhibits DNA synthesis.
(b) True   It is administered as an intravenous infusion in both immuno-
(c) True   competent and immunosuppressed patients.
(d) True
(e) False

317 **(a) False** – Associated with foscarnet
(b) False – Associated with ganciclovir which is indicated in severe CMV
infection in immunocompromised patients
(c) False – Associated with amphotericin
(d) True
(e) True

318 **(a) False**   Interferons are glycoproteins secreted by cells infected with
(b) True   viruses or foreign double-stranded DNA. They are non-
(c) True   antigenic and species specific.
(d) True
(e) False

319 Zidovudine (AZT):

   (a) Is licenced in the UK for the treatment of HIV-1 infection
   (b) Is administered by subcutaneous injection
   (c) Inhibits viral reverse transcription
   (d) Should be stopped if cotrimoxazole is required
   (e) Prolongs survival in late-stage AIDS

320 Adverse effects associated with AZT include:

   (a) Dose-dependent reticulocytopenia
   (b) Dose-dependent granulocytopenia
   (c) Nausea and vomiting
   (d) Cough
   (e) Blue-grey nail discoloration

321 The following are used to treat *Pneumocystis carinii* pneumonia (PCP) in patients with HIV infection:

   (a) Aztreonam
   (b) Intravenous co-trimoxazole
   (c) Ciprofloxacin
   (d) Pentamidine
   (e) Glucocorticoids if the arterial pO_2 is less than 60 mmHg

322 Chloroquine:

   (a) Only injures *Plasmodium* when the parasite is extracellular
   (b) Must be given by intravenous infusion in *P. vivax* malaria
   (c) Can cause irreversible visual loss when used as prolonged therapy
   (d) Should not be co-prescribed with proguanil
   (e) Is contraindicated in children under 10 years

323 The following acute *Plasmodium* infections are paired with their appropriate treatment:

   (a) Falciparum malaria in West Africa – quinine
   (b) Cerebral malaria in West Africa – quinine and chloroquine
   (c) *P. vivax* – chloroquine followed by primaquine
   (d) *P. vivax* in a pregnant woman – chloroquine, the primaquine being postponed until after delivery
   (e) Falciparum malaria in East Africa in a pregnant woman – halofantrine

324 Quinine sulfate:

   (a) Is the drug of choice in chloroquine-resistant falciparum malaria
   (b) Is available for intravenous and oral use
   (c) Is effective in eradicating the hepatic parasites in *P. vivax* malaria
   (d) Is contraindicated in renal failure
   (e) Large therapeutic doses cause tinnitus

319 (a) True   The exact role of AZT in the management of AIDS is
    (b) False   controversial. Specialist advice should be sought. It is
    (c) True   administered orally.
    (d) False
    (e) True

320 (a) True   AZT therapy is also associated with fatigue, headache,
    (b) True   insomnia and, more rarely, myopathy.
    (c) True
    (d) False
    (e) True

321 (a) False   High dose co-trimoxazole is first line standard treatment for
    (b) True   PCP in patients with HIV infection. After recovery, secondary
    (c) False   prophylaxis with oral co-trimoxazole is usual.
    (d) True
    (e) True

322 (a) False   Chloroquine is one of the most widely used antimalarial
    (b) False   drugs. Unfortunately the incidence of falciparum resistance to
    (c) True   chloroquine is becoming more widespread.
    (d) False
    (e) False

323 (a) True
    (b) False   – Quinine and chloroquine are antagonistic
    (c) True   – Primaquine is required to destroy the parasites in the liver and
                  prevent relapse
    (d) True   – After the standard course of chloroquine as for a non-pregnant
                  patient, chloroquine is continued weekly until delivery
    (e) False   – Falciparum malaria is particularly dangerous in the last trimester
                  – use quinine

324 (a) True   – If resistance is not a possibility, chloroquine may be used
    (b) True
    (c) False   – Primaquine
    (d) False
    (e) True   – Cinchonism, which also includes deafness, headache, nausea
                  and visual disturbance

325 The following adverse effects are paired with a causative antimalarial drug:

   (a) Lichenoid skin eruption − chloroquine
   (b) Stevens–Johnson syndrome − quinine
   (c) Hallucinations − mefloquine
   (d) Prolongation of QT_c halofantrine
   (e) Hemolytic anemia − primaquine

326 The following infections have been paired with appropriate drug therapy:

   (a) *Trypanosoma gambiense* (African sleeping sickness), early stages − pentamidine and suramin
   (b) Giardiasis − metronidazole
   (c) *Taenia saginata* (a tapeworm) − emetine
   (d) Threadworm − mebendazole
   (e) *Toxocara canis* − pyrantel

327 The following cytotoxic drugs are extremely emetogenic:

   (a) Cyclophosphamide
   (b) methotrexate
   (c) 5-fluorouracil
   (d) Mustine
   (e) Cisplatin

328 The following cytotoxic drugs may be associated with prolonged myelosup-pression:

   (a) Chlorambucil
   (b) Melphalan
   (c) BCNU (1,3-bis (2 chloroethyl-1-nitrourea))
   (d) Bleomycin
   (e) Vincristine

329 During cancer chemotherapy:

   (a) Infection is the commonest life-threatening complication
   (b) Infection is often acquired from the patient's own gut flora
   (c) If infection occurs, pyrexia is usually absent
   (d) Men and women must be strongly advised to avoid conception
   (e) There is a danger of inducing second malignancies

330 Cyclophosphamide:

   (a) Is normally used in combination with other cytotoxic agents
   (b) Is an alkylating agent
   (c) Causes granulocytopenia
   (d) Causes nausea and vomiting
   (e) Causes alopecia

325 (a) **True**
    (b) **False** – Recognized with pyrimethamine and sulfadoxine (Fansidar[R])
    (c) **True** – Also potentiates the bradycardic effect of β-blockers
    (d) **True**
    (e) **True** – In glucose 6-phosphate dehydrogenase deficient patients

326 (a) **True**
    (b) **True**
    (c) **False** – A single dose of praziquantel is curative
    (d) **True** – Pyrantel also effective
    (e) **False** – Diethylcarbamazine, corticosteroids may be needed to treat
    allergic reactions to dying larvae

327 (a) **True**   Nausea and vomiting are often the principal immediate toxic
    (b) **False**   effects associated with cytotoxic chemotherapy. To avoid
    (c) **False**   tissue necrosis, another immediate effect, expert
    (d) **True**   attention to vascular access is mandatory.
    (e) **True**

328 (a) **True**   There are two patterns of bone marrow recovery after
    (b) **True**   suppression (*CPT*, Fig 45.7), rapid and delayed. Vincristine
    (c) **True**   and bleomycin seldom cause myelosuppression.
    (d) **False**
    (e) **False**

329 (a) **True**   Broad-spectrum antibacterial treatment must be started
    (b) **True**   empirically in febrile neutropenic patients without waiting for
    (c) **False**   culture results. The effect on fertility and the risk of future
    (d) **True**   fetal abnormalities are very variable Alkylating agents are
    (e) **True**   particularly harmful. Successful pregnancies are not unusual
    in women at least 6 months after completion of chemother
    apy. Sperm storage should be considered.

330 (a) **True**   Cyclophosphamide is most useful in the treatment of various
    (b) **True**   lymphomas and leukemias and in myeloma but it also has
    (c) **True**   some effect in other malignancies (e.g. breast cancer, small
    (d) **True**   cell lung cancer). It may be given by mouth or intravenous
    (e) **True**   injection.

331 Sterile hemorrhagic cystitis is associated with:

(a) Cyclophosphamide
(b) Ifosfamide
(c) Acrolein
(d) Corticosteroids
(e) Mesna

332 Methotrexate:

(a) Is a folinic acid antagonist
(b) The toxicity of high doses can be reduced by giving folinic acid 24 hours after the methotrexate
(c) Doses should be reduced if allopurinol is administered
(d) Chronic treatment can cause cirrhosis
(e) Is the treatment of choice for choriocarcinoma

333 The following cytotoxic drugs are paired with a characteristic adverse effect:

(a) Doxorubicin – peripheral neuropathy
(b) Etoposide – alopecia
(c) Daunorubicin – cardiomyopathy
(d) Methotrexate – oral ulceration
(e) 6-mercaptopurine – pulmonary fibrosis

334 During cisplatin therapy:

(a) Pretreatment hydration is mandatory
(b) Pretreatment with ondansetron reduces the nausea and vomiting
(c) Visual disturbances are common
(d) Magnesium supplements are usually given
(e) Hepatotoxicity is dose related and dose limiting

335 Recombinant human erythropoietin is used to treat:

(a) Iron deficient anemia when iron is malabsorbed
(b) Pernicious anemia
(c) Anemia of chronic renal failure
(d) AZT-induced anemia
(e) Clozapine-induced agranulocytosis

336 Filgrastim (human granulocyte colony stimulating factor):

(a) Is usually administered by subcutaneous injection
(b) Causes immediate transient neutropenia
(c) Is used in myeloid leukemia
(d) Stimulates proliferation and differentiation of progenitor cells of all granulocyte lines
(e) Causes bone pain

331 (a) **True**   Mesna protects the urinary tract against the irritant metabolites
    (b) **True**   of cyclophosphamide and ifosfamide and in particular
    (c) **True**   acrolein, a metabolite of these agents.
    (d) **False**
    (e) **False**

332 (a) **True**
    (b) **True**
    (c) **False** – Allopurinol antagonizes methotrexate by increasing purine
                 availability
    (d) **True**
    (e) **True**

333 (a) **False** – Peripheral neuropathy is common with vincristine
    (b) **True** – Etoposide is particularly active in small cell lung cancer
    (c) **True**
    (d) **True**
    (e) **False** – Pulmonary fibrosis is associated with busulphan therapy

334 (a) **True**
    (b) **True**
    (c) **False** – Ototoxicity develops in up to 30% of patients
    (d) **True**
    (e) **False** – Nephrotoxicity occurs

335 (a) **False** – Use parenteral iron
    (b) **False** – Use parenteral vitamin B_{12}
    (c) **True**
    (d) **True**
    (e) **False**

336 (a) **True** – Often self-administered
    (b) **True**
    (c) **False** – Increases proliferation of the malignant clone
    (d) **True**
    (e) **True** – Also myalgia, fever, splenomegaly, thrombocytopenia and
                abnormal liver enzymes

9 CLINICAL IMMUNOPHARMACOLOGY

337 Azathioprine:

   (a) Is metabolized to 6-mercaptopurine
   (b) Inhibits delayed hypersensitivity (cell mediated immunity) and those aspects of inflammation that require cell division
   (c) Is administered by subcutaneous injection
   (d) Causes bone marrow suppression
   (e) Concurrent allopurinol increases the clearance of azathioprine

338 Cyclophosphamide is used for its immunosuppressive action in the following indications:

   (a) Cystic fibrosis
   (b) Autoimmune thrombocytopenia
   (c) Nephrotic syndrome with minimal microscopic glomerular changes
   (d) Nephritis due to systemic lupus erythematosus
   (e) Wegener's granulomatosis

339 Glucocorticoids inhibit:

   (a) Platelet thromboxane A_2 synthesis
   (b) Histamine release
   (c) Leukotriene LTD_4 synthesis
   (d) Neutrophil production
   (e) Lipocortin synthesis

340 The following agents are used to treat graft-versus-host disease:

   (a) Glucocorticoids
   (b) Cyclosporin
   (c) OKT3 antibodies
   (d) Foscarnet
   (e) Ganciclovir

341 Adverse effects associated with cyclosporin include:

   (a) Nephrotoxicity
   (b) Nausea and gastrointestinal disturbances
   (c) Alopecia
   (d) Tremor
   (e) Hypokalemia

342 The following are indicated in the management of acute anaphylactic shock following a bee sting out of hospital and without monitoring facilities:

   (a) Intramuscular adrenaline (0.5–1 ml, 1 in 1000)
   (b) Intravenous adrenaline (10 ml, 1 in 10 000)
   (c) Intravenous hydrocortisone
   (d) Intravenous chlorpromazine
   (e) Oxygen

337 **(a) True** Azathioprine is an antimetabolite and therefore most
(b) True effective on proliferating cells. It is administered by mouth.
(c) False It is used to prevent transplant rejection and with some
(d) True success in the treatment of autoimmune diseases such as
(e) False systemic lupus erythematosus and chronic active hepatitis.
Owing to its potential toxicity (bone marrow) it is usually
reserved for situations in which corticosteroids alone are
inadequate.

338 **(a) False** Cyclophosphamide, in addition to its uses in oncology as a
(b) False cytotoxic drug, is particularly valuable in aggressive auto-
(c) True immune diseases by inhibiting lymphocyte proliferation.
(d) True
(e) True

339 **(a) False** Glucocorticoids stimulate lipocortin synthesis and inhibit
(b) True type I, II, III and IV hypersensitivity reactions. They are the
(c) True most widely used immunosuppressive agents. They inhibit
(d) False eicosanoid synthesis in nucleated cells and increase the
(e) False neutrophil count in peripheral blood.

340 **(a) True**
(b) True – Specific T lymphocyte suppressor, primarily the T-helper cells
(c) True
(d) False – Anti-CMV
(e) False – Anti-CMV

341 **(a) True**
(b) True – In up to 20% of patients
(c) False – Hirsutism
(d) False – May be an early sign of toxic plasma concentration
(e) False – Hyperkalemia

342 **(a) True** – Life saving
(b) False – May induce ventricular fibrillation
(c) True – But takes 4–6 hours to be of benefit
(d) False – The use of intravenous antihistamines is controversial
(e) True – Intravenous fluids (e.g. hemacel, also of value and may be
available in an ambulance. The use of intravenous anti-
histaminer is controversial).

343 Terfenadine:

(a) Is a H_1-receptor antagonist
(b) Is used as a sedative in children
(c) Is an effective antiemetic
(d) Is used prophylactically in hayfever
(e) Plasma concentration is increased by co-administration of erythromycin

344 The following are used in the management of allergic rhinitis (hayfever):

(a) Oral H_1-receptor antagonist
(b) Oral theophylline
(c) Nasal cromoglycate
(d) Nasal salbutamol
(e) Nasal corticosteroids

345 Most children should have received the following vaccines before entry into primary school:

(a) Measles, mumps and rubella
(b) Influenza
(c) Diphtheria, tetanus and pertussis
(d) Polio
(e) Smallpox

343 **(a) True**   Terfenadine, astemizole, cetirizine and loratadine are
    (b) False   "non-sedative" antihistamines.
    (c) False
    (d) True
    (e) True – This combination may induce ventricular tachycardia

344 **(a) True**   Avoidance of allergens is ideal but rarely practical. With the
    (b) False   exception of oral H_1-blockers, local therapy is preferred.
    (c) True
    (d) False
    (e) True

345 **(a) True**   Live vaccines should be avoided in the immunosuppressed.
    (b) False   Menningococcal vaccines are now available during epidemics
    (c) True   and for travelers going into areas of high incidence of
    (d) True   meningococcal carriage. *Haemophilus influenzae* b vaccine
    (e) False   is administered during the second year of life.

10 THE SKIN

346 The following are effective in the management of acne:
- (a) Topical retinoic acid
- (b) Topical podophyllin
- (c) Topical triamcinolone
- (d) Topical cold tar
- (e) Oral tetracycline

347 Isotretinoin:
- (a) Is a synthetic vitamin D analog
- (b) The usual course is 2 weeks
- (c) Is teratogenic
- (d) Causes hirsutism
- (e) Is eliminated over a period of weeks

348 The following are of value in the management of eczema:
- (a) Topical corticosteroids
- (b) Topical gamolenic acid
- (c) Dithranol
- (d) Calcipotriol
- (e) Emulsifying ointment

349 Local application of the following are of benefit in the management of psoriasis:
- (a) Acitretin
- (b) Salicylic acid
- (c) Psoralens
- (d) Dithranol
- (e) Calcipotriol

350 Calcipotriol:
- (a) Is present in evening primrose oil
- (b) Is a derivative of calcitonin
- (c) Causes marked erythema if applied to normal skin
- (d) Causes yellow discoloration of the skin but not sclerae
- (e) Causes hypercalcemia

351 The following infections/infestations are paired with an appropriate treatment:
- (a) *Candida* vulvovaginitis – topical ketoconazole
- (b) Fungal nail infections – oral griseofulvin
- (c) *Tinea corporis* – topical clotrimazole
- (d) Initial or recurrent genital herpes simplex – oral acyclovir
- (e) Scabies – lindane

346 (a) **True** Acne vulgaris occurs in at least 90% of adolescents. The
    (b) **False** topical use of peeling agents such as benzoyl peroxide or
    (c) **False** retinoic acid on a regular basis is usually all that is necessary.
    (d) **False** In more severe cases oral anti-bacterial drugs are beneficial
    (e) **True** and if this is ineffective oral isotretinoin may be considered by
           specialists.

347 (a) **False** – Isotretinoin is a vitamin A analog
    (b) **False** – Prescribed under hospital supervision usually for 2 months
    (c) **True**
    (d) **False**
    (e) **True** – Persistent risk of teratogenicity for at least 1 month after
           stopping oral therapy

348 (a) **True** If the eczema is wet the topical use of drying agents such as
    (b) **False** lotions of aluminum acetate or calamine are useful. When the
    (c) **False** lesions are dry and scaly the use of moisturising cream (e.g.
    (d) **False** E45) combined with a keratolytic is beneficial. Topical corti-
    (e) **True** costeroids are often required. Nocturnal pruritus may be
           relieved by sedative antihistamines.

349 (a) **False** – Acitretin is an oral retinoid used in severe, resistant or
           complicated psoriasis
    (b) **True** – Enhances rate of loss of surface scale
    (c) **False** – PUVA (photochemotherapy using an oral psoralen with long
           wave ultraviolet radiation) is an effective but unlicensed treat-
           ment for psoriasis
    (d) **True** – Irritates normal skin
    (e) **True** – Does not irritate normal skin

350 (a) **False**
    (b) **False** – Calcipotriol is a derivative of vitamin D
    (c) **False**
    (d) **False** – Occurs with excess β-carotene in diet which may be confused
           with jaundice, differentiated by normal sclerae
    (e) **True** – Associated with excessive application

351 (a) **True** With unusual/recurrent skin infections consider diabetes/
    (b) **True** immunosuppression.
    (c) **True**
    (d) **True**
    (e) **True**

11 CLINICAL TOXICOLOGY

352 Methadone:

(a) Has the potential to cause dependence
(b) Can only be prescribed to registered addicts by doctors with a special license
(c) Is usually administered as an elixir
(d) Depresses the cough center
(e) Effects are reversed by naloxone

353 The following are clinical signs consistent with heroin (diamorphine) intoxication:

(a) Hypertension
(b) Rapid respiratory rate
(c) Hypothermia
(d) Pin-point pupils
(e) Slurred speech

354 Features of the opioid withdrawal syndrome include:

(a) Yawning
(b) Rhinorrhea
(c) Mydriasis
(d) Diarrhea
(e) Tremor

355 Specific causes of death which are positively related to smoking include:

(a) Ischemic heart disease
(b) Cancer of the esophagus
(c) Emphysema
(d) Aortic aneurysm
(e) Cancer of the tongue

356 There is an increased rate of metabolism of the following drugs in smokers:

(a) Diazepam
(b) Phenytoin
(c) Ethanol
(d) Warfarin
(e) Theophylline

357 Ethyl alcohol (ethanol):

(a) The majority of oral ethanol is absorbed from the small intestine
(b) Ethanol delays gastic emptying
(c) 95% of ingested ethanol is metabolized
(d) Ethanol elimination demonstrates first order kinetics
(e) Is second to heroin as the most important drug of dependence in Western Europe

352 **(a) True**   Methadone elixir/mixture is the mainstay of many drug
    (b) False   addiction clinics. It has a long half-life of 15–55 hours and it is
    (c) True   very difficult to administer these oral formulations as an
    (d) True   injection.
    (e) True

353 **(a) False**   Initially intravenous heroin produces an intense euphoria for
    (b) False   several seconds (often accompanied by nausea/vomiting).
    (c) True   Many chronic users often claim the only effect is remission
    (d) True   from abstinence symptoms.
    (e) True

354 **(a) True**   Withdrawal symptoms generally start at the time the next dose
    (b) True   would usually be given and their intensity is related to the
    (c) True   usual dose. For heroin, symptoms usually reach a maximum
    (d) True   at 36–72 hours and gradually subside over the next 5–10
    (e) True   days.

355 **(a) True**   In the UK, in men under 70 years, the ratio of death rate
    (b) True   among cigarette smokers to non-smokers is 2:1.
    (c) True
    (d) True
    (e) True

356 **(a) False**   In addition to pharmacokinetic differences, smokers may
    (b) False   exhibit altered pharmacodynamic responses (e.g. smokers
    (c) False   show less CNS depression after a standard dose of
    (d) False   diazepam than non-smokers).
    (e) True

357 **(a) True**   It has been estimated that the incidence of alcoholism in
    (b) True   North America and Western Europe is nearly 5% of the
    (c) True   population. Ethanol is a weak enzyme inducer and differences
    (d) False   in rate of ethanol metabolism are principally genetic.
    (e) False

358 Cardiovascular complications associated with alcohol consumption include:

  (a) Atrial fibrillation
  (b) Buerger's disease
  (c) Cardiomyopathy
  (d) Coronary artery disease
  (e) Peripheral vascular disease

359 Delirium tremens:

  (a) Occurs in approximately 60% of patients withdrawing from alcohol
  (b) Has a mortality of 5–10%
  (c) Benzodiazepines are contraindicated
  (d) Thiamine should be administered parenterally
  (e) Phenytoin should be administered prophylactically to prevent convulsions

360 Chronic use of anabolic steroids is associated with:

  (a) Pancreatitis
  (b) Ototoxicity
  (c) Hepatic tumors
  (d) Cardiomyopathy
  (e) Peripheral neuropathy

361 The combination of coma, dilated pupils, hyperreflexia and tachycardia is consistent with overdose of the following drugs when taken alone:

  (a) Co-proxamol
  (b) Dothiepin
  (c) Aspirin
  (d) Amitriptyline
  (e) Lorazepam

358 **(a) True**
    (b) False – Associated with smoking
    (c) True
    (d) False – Associated with smoking
    (e) False – Associated with smoking

359 **(a) False** – < 10%
    (b) True
    (c) False – Chlormethiazole and benzodiazepines (long half-life) are suitable sedatives
    (d) True – To avoid precipitation of acute thiamine deficiency when intravenous dextrose/oral carbohydrates are administered
    (e) False

360 **(a) False**   Anabolic steroids are abused by athletes to build up muscle
    (b) False   tissue.
    (c) True
    (d) True
    (e) False

361 **(a) False**   A meticulous, rapid but thorough clinical examination is
    (b) True   essential not only to exclude other causes of coma/abnormal
    (c) False   behavior, but also because the symptoms and signs may be
    (d) True   characteristic of certain poisons.
    (e) False

Table 3 Clinical manifestations of some common poisons.

Symptoms/signs of acute overdose	Common poisons
Coma, hypotension, flaccidity	Benzodiazepines and other hypnosedatives, alcohol.
Coma, pin-point pupils, hypoventilation	Opioids
Coma, dilated pupils, hyperreflexia, tachycardi(a)	Tricyclic antidepressants, phenothiazines; other drugs with anticholinergic properties
Restlessness, hypertonia, hyperreflexia pyrexia	Amphetamines, MDMA, anticholinergic agents.
Convulsions	Tricyclic antidepressants, phenothiazines, carbon monoxide, monoamine oxidase inhibitors, mefenamic acid, theophylline, hypoglycemic agents, lithium, cyanide
Tinnitus, overbreathing, pyrexia, sweating, flushing, usually alert	Salicylates.
Burns in mouth, dysphagia, abdominal pain	Corrosives, caustics, paraquat.

362 The following suspected overdoses are indications for emergency measurement of drug concentration:

  (a) Iron
  (b) Methanol
  (c) Amitriptyline
  (d) Temazepam
  (e) Salicylates

363 Alkaline diuresis enhances the elimination of:

  (a) Amphetamine
  (b) Salicylates
  (c) Theophylline
  (d) Phenobarbitone
  (e) Dothiepin

362 (a) **True**
    (b) **True**
    (c) **False**
    (d) **False**
    (e) **True**

Table 4 Common indications for emergency measurements of drug concentration.

Suspected overdose	Effect on management
Paracetamol	Administration of antidotes – acetylcysteine or methionine
Iron	Administration of antidote – desferrioxamine
Methanol/ethylene glycol	Administration of antidote – ethanol ± dialysis
Lithium	Dialysis
Salicylates	Simple rehydration or alkaline diuresis or dialysis
Theophylline	Necessity of ITU admission

363 (a) **False**   Methods to increase poison elimination are appropriate in less
    (b) **True**   than 5% of overdose causes.
    (c) **False**
    (d) **True**
    (e) **False**

Table 5 Methods and indications for enhancement of poison elimination

Metho(d)	Poison
Alkaline diuresis	Salicylates, phenobarbitone
Acid diuresis	Phencyclidine, ?amphetamine
Hemodialysis (peritoneal dialysis is also effective but two to three times less efficient)	Salicylates, methanol, ethylene glycol, lithium, phenobarbitone
Charcoal hemoperfusion (rarely necessary)	Barbiturates, theophylline disopyramide
"Gastrointestinal dialysis" using activated charcoal	Salicylates, most anticonvulsants, digoxin, theophylline, quinine

364 The following poisons/drugs have been correctly paired with an appropriate antidote/specific measure:

(a) Paracetamol – acetylcysteine
(b) Iron – desferrioxamine
(c) Dextropropoxyphene – naloxone
(d) Organophosphorus insecticides – dicobalt edatate
(e) Methanol – ethanol

364 (a) **True**
    (b) **True**
    (c) **True**
    (d) **False**
    (e) **True**

Table 6 Antidotes and other specific measures.

Overdose drug	Antidote/other specific measures
Paracetamol	Acetylcysteine i.v. Methionine p°.
Iron	Desferrioxamine
Cyanide	Oxygen, amyl nitrate (inhalation), dicobalt edetate i.v., sodium nitrate i.v., followed by sodium thiosulphate i.v.
Benzodiazepines	Flumazenil i.v.
β-Blocker	Glucagon Atropine Isoprenaline
Carbon monoxide	Oxygen Hyperbaric oxygen
Methanol/ethylene glycol	Ethanol
Lead	Sodium calcium edetate i.v. Penicillamine p°. Dimercaptosuccinic acid (DMSA) i.v. or p°.
Mercury	Dimercaptopropane sulfonate (DMPS) Dimercaptosuccinic acid (DMSA) Dimercaprol Penicillamine
Opioids	Naloxone
Organophosphorus insecticides	Atropine, pralidoxime
Digoxin	Digoxin specific fab antibody fragments
Calcium channel blockers	Calcium chloride or gluconate i.v. glucagon
Insulin	50% dextrose i.v. glucagon i.v. or i.m.

*NB: DMSA and DMPS are not licensed in the UK.
    Advice should be sought from a Poisons Information Centre.

365 An 18-year-old woman is admitted 2 hours after taking 50 paracetamol and 50 aspirin tablets. The following statements are correct:

  (a) She is likely to be in a grade IV coma
  (b) Stomach washout is indicated
  (c) Acetylcysteine should be administered
  (d) Blood gases are likely to show a mixed metabolic acidosis/respiratory alkalosis
  (e) If the prothrombin time is prolonged acetylcysteine is contraindicated

366 Medical practitioners have an obligation to notify the Home Office of addicts whom they believe to be taking any of the following drugs:

  (a) Diamorphine
  (b) Dipipanone
  (c) Phenobarbitone
  (d) LSD
  (e) Cocaine

367 The following are confirmed aphrodisiacs:

  (a) Ginseng
  (b) Oysters
  (c) Extract of rhino horn
  (d) Passion fruit
  (e) Vitamin E

365 **(a) False**   Paracetamol and salicylate overdoses only very rarely
    (b) True   cause coma acutely. Salicylate overdose is an indication
    (c) True   for late stomach washout (some authorities disagree).
    (d) True
    (e) False

366 **(a) True**   Notification must be made within 7 days to the Chief Medical
    (b) True   Officer at the Home Office giving name, sex, date of birth,
    (c) False   address and NHS number together with the drug involved,
    (d) False   whether the patient injects any drug (whether or not
    (e) True   notifiable) and the date of attendance. Notification is not
                necessary if the doctor believes that the drug is medically
                necessary or if the doctor or a colleague has notified the
                patient within the preceding 12 months.

367 **(a) False**   The authors recommend champagne.
    (b) False
    (c) False
    (d) False
    (e) False

12 PRACTICE MCQ EXAMINATION

Mark +2 for a correct response, 0 for no response and −1 for an incorrect response. 50% is the pass mark for the examination (i.e. 300/600 score marks). Allow 90 minutes in one sitting to complete the examination.

1   The following receptors have been paired correctly with their agonist:

(a) β_1-receptor – salbutamol
(b) β_2-receptor – terbutaline
(c) α-receptor – noradrenaline
(d) 5-HT$_{1D}$ receptors – sumatriptan
(e) Dopamine D$_2$-receptors – chlorpromazine

2   The following decrease the rate of gastric emptying and hence the rate of oral drug absorption:

(a) Amitriptyline
(b) Duodenal ulcer
(c) Paracetamol
(d) Migraine
(e) Metoclopramide

3   A "normal" 75-year-old man will eliminate the following drugs more slowly than a "normal" 25-year-old:

(a) Gentamicin
(b) Digoxin
(c) Chlorpropamide
(d) Atenolol
(e) Ciprofloxacin

4   The metabolism of the following drugs can be saturated within the usual dose range:

(a) Paracetamol
(b) Gentamicin
(c) Heparin
(d) Alcohol
(e) Phenytoin

5   The elimination half-life of the following drugs is greater than 12 hours:

(a) Heparin
(b) Adenosine
(c) Etridronate
(d) Fluoxetine
(e) Azithromycin

6   The following drugs block reuptake of 5-hydroxytryptamine:

(a) Buspirone
(b) Diazepam
(c) Pizotifen
(d) Ondansetron
(e) Fluoxetine

1 **(a) False** – Salbutamol is a β_2-agonist
   (b) True
   (c) True
   (d) True – Sumatriptan is used to treat migraine
   (e) False – Most antipsychotic drugs are D_2-antagonists

2 **(a) True** – Anticholinergic action
   (b) False
   (c) False
   (d) True – Hence the rationale for combining metaclopramide with minor
   analgesics in migraine
   (e) False

3 **(a) True**   Glomerular filtration rate decreases with age. See *CPT*,
   (b) True   Chapter 10, p.88.
   (c) True
   (d) True
   (e) True

4 **(a) False**   For drugs that exhibit saturation kinetics a small increase in
   (b) False   dose can lead to a disproportionate increase in plasma
   (c) True   concentration.
   (d) True
   (e) True

5 **(a) False** – 0.5–2.5 hours
   (b) False – A few seconds
   (c) True
   (d) True – Approximately 2 days
   (e) True

6 **(a) False** – Partial agonist
   (b) False
   (c) False – $5\text{-}HT_{1+2}$ antagonist (migraine prophylaxis)
   (d) False – $5\text{-}HT_3$ antagonist
   (e) True – Antidepressant

7   Individuals who are categorized as slow acetylators (i.e. have a relatively low activity of hepatic N-acetyltransferase):

(a) Have a prevalence of 5–10% in Caucasians in the UK
(b) Are more likely to develop thrombocytopenia, nephrotic syndrome and rash during gold treatment
(c) Are more likely to develop hepatotoxicity following halothane anesthesia
(d) Are more likely to develop antinuclear antibodies during hydralazine therapy
(e) Are more likely to develop peripheral neuropathy during isoniazid therapy

8   The following drugs are confirmed teratogens in man:

(a) Phenytoin
(b) Retinoids
(c) Salbutamol
(d) Erythromycin
(e) Folic acid

9   Which of the following is generally suitable for the management of lower urinary tract infection diagnosed during pregnancy:

(a) Amoxycillin
(b) Cefadroxil
(c) Aztreonam
(d) Co-trimoxazole
(e) Ciprofloxacin

7 (a) False
   (b) False
   (c) False
   (d) True
   (e) True

Table 7 Variations in drug metabolism due to genetic polymorphism.

Pharmacogenetic variation	Drugs involved	Mechanism	Inheritance	Occurrence
Rapid acetylator status	Increased hepatic N-acetyltransferase	Autosomal dominant	40% whites	Isoniazid; hydralazine; some sulfonamides; phenelzine; dapsone procainamide
Suxamethonium sensitivity	Several types of abnormal plasma pseudocholinesterase	Autosomal recessive	Most common form 1:2500	Suxamethonium
Defective hydroxylation of debrisoquine	Functionally defective cytochrome $P_{450}2D6$	Autosomal recessive	8% Britons; 1% Saudi Arabians; 30% Chinese Orientals	Debrisoquine; metoprolol perhexiline; nortriptyline
Ethanol sensitivity	Relatively low rate of alcohol metabolism	Usual in some ethnic groups	Orientals	Alcohol

8 (a) True
   (b) True
   (c) False
   (d) False
   (e) False

Table 8 Some drugs that are definitely teratogenic in humans

Thalidomide	Androgens
Cytoxic agents	Progestogens
Alcohol	Diethylstilbestrol
Warfarin	Radioisotopes
Retinoids	Some live vaccines
Most anticonvulsants	Lithium

Some drugs e.g. misoprostol, ergotamine can cause abortion.

9 (a) True   Urinary tract infection in pregnancy should be treated
   (b) True   without delay to prevent progression to pyelonephritis.
   (c) False
   (d) False
   (e) False

10 Tricyclic antidepressants such as imipramine and amitriptyline:
(a) May cause anticholinergic side effects
(b) May cause postural hypotension
(c) May cause broadening of the QRS in overdose
(d) Have been shown to be less effective in endogenous depression than newer antidepressants such as mianserin and lofepramine
(e) Should be stopped at least 2 weeks before electroconvulsive therapy

11 Carbidopa when administered with levodopa:
(a) Inhibits the intracerebral metabolism of levodopa
(b) Reduces nausea by permitting a lower dose of levodopa
(c) Reduces postural hypotension by permitting a lower dose of levodopa
(d) Delays the onset of therapeutic effect
(e) Abolishes the "on-off" phenomenon

12 Carbamazepine:
(a) Is a benzodiazepine
(b) Induces its own metabolism
(c) Is a GABA antagonist
(d) Is contraindicated in patients with ischemic heart disease
(e) May cause hyponatremia

13 It is rational and common practice to commence treatment with the following drugs with a loading dose:
(a) Levodopa
(b) Captopril
(c) Amiodarone
(d) Carbamazepine
(e) Salbutamol

14 Captopril has the following properties:
(a) Inhibits conversion of renin to angiotensin
(b) Inhibits the destruction of bradykinin
(c) Increases urinary elimination of potassium
(d) Can be used as a mixed arterial and venous dilator in heart failure
(e) Combination with thiazide diuretics is contraindicated

15 A man is admitted within 3 hours of the onset of chest pain. His ECG is consistent with an acute myocardial infarction. Streptokinase should not be administered if:
(a) The patient is over 70 years old
(b) The patient had a stroke due to a cerebral hemorrhage 3 months previously
(c) The patient is already taking atenolol for hypertension (average blood pressure on treatment of 150/95)
(d) The patient has asthma
(e) The patient was given streptokinase 3 months previously following a myocardial infarction

10 **(a) True**   Although toxic in overdose, associated with adverse effects
    (b) True   and with a delay in onset of therapeutic action the traditional
    (c) True   tricyclic antidepressants are still regarded by many as first line
    (d) False   treatment in most patients with endogenous depression.
    (e) False

11 **(a) False**   Carbidopa, a peripheral dopa decarboxylase inhibitor, inhibits
    (b) True   the extracerebral metabolism of the levodopa to dopamine.
    (c) True
    (d) False
    (e) False

12 **(a) False**   Carbamazepine is an effective anticonvulsant which is used in
    (b) True   all forms of epilepsy except absence seizures.
    (c) False
    (d) False
    (e) True

13 **(a) False**
    (b) False
    (c) True
    (d) False
    (e) False

14 **(a) False** – Inhibits angiotensin I conversion to angiotensin II
    (b) True – May be the cause of cough
    (c) False – Can cause hyperkalemia
    (d) True
    (e) False – Often necessary in hypertension and heart failure. If already on
                    a diuretic beware first dose hypotension

15 **(a) False** – Even greater reduction in mortality
    (b) True
    (c) False
    (d) False
    (e) True – Give tissue plasminogen activator

16 The following agents may be used in the long term treatment of chronic atrial fibrillation in a 55-year-old female:

(a) Mexiletine
(b) Warfarin
(c) Adenosine
(d) Sotalol
(e) Verapamil

17 Estimation of plasma/serum drug concentrations are useful in controlling the dose required of:

(a) Diclofenac
(b) Omeprazole
(c) Lithium carbonate
(d) Flupenthixol decanoate
(e) Cyclosporin

18 The following antiarrythmic treatments are correctly paired with an appropriate indication:

(a) Digoxin – rapid atrial fibrillation
(b) Verapamil – atrial fibrillation complicating WPW
(c) Lignocaine – ventricular tachycardia
(d) Atropine – symptomatic bradycardia post myocardial infarction
(e) Demand pacemaker – first degree heart block

19 Heparin:

(a) Is contraindicated in unstable angina
(b) Is monitored by measurement of the prothrombin time
(c) Is much less effective in antithrombin III deficiency
(d) Is reversed by vitamin K
(e) Is indicated in the long-term management of chronic atrial fibrillation

20 The following drugs are associated with a decreased clearance of theophylline:

(a) Cimetidine
(b) Erythromycin
(c) Ciprofloxacin
(d) Phenytoin
(e) Rifampicin

21 The following are indicated in acute severe asthma in a boy of 12 years:

(a) High concentration oxygen
(b) Nebulized salbutamol
(c) Intravenous hydrocortisone
(d) Intravenous isoprenaline
(e) Intravenous crystalloid

22 The following drugs reduce gastric acid secretion:

(a) Sucralfate
(b) Cimetidine
(c) Salbutamol
(d) Cisapride
(e) Bismuth

16 **(a) False** – A Class I antiarrhythmic drug
    (b) True – Reduces the risk of embolism
    (c) False – Used in the diagnosis and immediate treatment of SVT
    (d) True – A β–blocker with additional Class III antiarrhythmic activity
    (e) True – A calcium channel blocker

17 **(a) False** – Diclofenac is a non-steroidal anti-inflammatory drug
    (b) False – Omeprazole inhibits gastric acid production
    (c) True – In addition to serum concentrations thyroid function should be monitored
    (d) False – Pimozide is used to treat schizophrenia. Cardiac arrhythmias have been reported and an ECG should be performed before starting theraphy and periodically at doses over 16mg daily.
    (e) True – Cyclosporin is a potent immunosuppressant which is of particular value in organ transplantation. It has little effect on the bone marrow but is nephrotoxic. There is considerable interindividual variability in its pharmacokinetics

18 **(a) True** – NB: cardioversion is often effective in acute AF
    (b) False – May increase ventricular rate
    (c) True
    (d) True
    (e) False – No therapy indicated

19 **(a) False** – Routine treatment
    (b) False – Intravenous infusions monitored by APTT
    (c) True – Binding to antithrombin III is a major action
    (d) False – Reversed by protamine sulfate
    (e) False – Warfarin is more practical in chronic therapy to reduce the risk of thromboembolism

20 **(a) True**   Through inhibition of hepatic enzymes. Theophylline has a
    (b) True   narrow therapeutic index hence such interactions are clinically
    (c) True   significant.
    (d) False
    (e) False

21 **(a) True**   The increasing mortality of acute severe asthma is partially
    (b) True   due to failure to recognize the severity of an exacerbation and
    (c) True   delayed use of corticosteroids.
    (d) False
    (e) True

22 **(a) False** – A complex of aluminum hydroxide and sulfated sucrose
    (b) True – An H_2-blocker
    (c) False – A β_2-agonist
    (d) False – A motility stimulant used in non-ulcer dyspepsia, esophageal reflux and gastric stasis
    (e) False – Stimulates mucosal protective prostaglandin, bicarbonate secretion and has a direct toxic effect on *Helicobacter pylori*

23 Omeprazole:

   (a) Blocks the hydrogen–potassium adenosine triphosphatase enzyme system

   (b) Is a synthetic analog of prostaglandin E

   (c) Blackens the tongue

   (d) Is an effective treatment for peptic ulcer

   (e) Is indicated for reflux esophagitis

24 The following are associated with dose-dependent hepatotoxicity:

   (a) Paracetamol

   (b) Halothane

   (c) Methotrexate

   (d) Chlorpromazine

   (e) Erythromycin lactobionate

25 The following drugs should be avoided in patients with liver disease who are jaundiced with ascites:

   (a) Diazepam

   (b) Spironolactone

   (c) Magnesium trisilicate mixture

   (d) Indomethacin

   (e) Metronidazole

23 **(a) True**
    (b) False – Misoprostol is a synthetic prostaglandin analog
    (c) False – Bismuth blackens the tongue
    (d) True
    (e) True

24 **(a) True**
    (b) False
    (c) True
    (d) False
    (e) False

Table 9 Dose-dependent hepatotoxicity

Drug	Mechanism	Comment/predisposing factors
Paracetamol	Hepatitis	See Chapter 50
Salicylates	Focal hepatocellular necrosis	Autoimmune disease (especially SLE)
	Reye's syndrome	In children – viral infection
Tetracycline	Central and mid-zonal necrosis with fat droplets	
Azathioprine	Cholestasis + hepatitis	Underlying liver disease
Methotrexate	Hepatic fibrosis	
Fusidic acid	Cholestasis, conjugated hyperbilirubinemi(a)	Rare
Rifampicin	Cholestasis, mixed conjugated and unconjugated hyperbilirubinemia	Transient
Synthetic estrogens	Cholestasis, may precipitate gall stones	Underlying liver disease rare now low-dose estrogens are generally given
HMGCoA reductase inhibitors	Unknown	Usually mild and asymptomatic

SLE Systemic lupus erythematosus.

25 **(a) True** – Can precipitate coma
    (b) False – Aldosterone antagonist useful in treatment of edema in hepatic failure
    (c) False
    (d) True – Increased risk of gastrointestinal bleeding and fluid retention
    (e) False

26 Which of the following antibacterial drugs would be appropriate in a 3-year-old child with acute otitis media who has a history of penicillin allergy?

(a) Amoxycillin
(b) Doxycycline
(c) Erythromycin
(d) Ciprofloxacin
(e) Gentamicin

27 The following treatment is appropriate for the indication named:

(a) *Campylobacter* enteritis – erythromycin
(b) Typhoid fever – ciprofloxacin
(c) Meningococcal meningitis – benzylpenicillin
(d) Herpes simplex encephalitis – acyclovir
(e) Threadworm infection in a child >2 years – mebendazole

28 Treatment with an intravenous aminoglycoside (e.g. gentamicin):

(a) Is contraindicated in neonatal septicemia
(b) Is useful for anaerobic infections
(c) Is relatively contraindicated in myasthenia gravis
(d) Is associated with ototoxicity which is usually irreversible
(e) Is contraindicated in cystic fibrosis

29 The following drugs have been correctly paired with an associated adverse effect:

(a) Cisplatin – severe nausea and vomiting
(b) Cimetidine – gastric carcinoma
(c) Clindamycin – pseudomembranous colitis
(d) Interferon α – Kaposi's sarcoma
(e) Doxorubicin – cardiomyopathy

30 The first line treatment of pulmonary TB in the UK in an immunocompetent patient includes an initial phase of 2 months treatment with:

(a) Isoniazid
(b) Rifampicin
(c) Pyrazinamide
(d) Ethambutol
(e) Streptomycin

31 A 25-year-old pregnant woman who was using chloroquine as malaria prophylaxis returns to the UK with cerebral malaria. The woman is 27 weeks pregnant. The following are appropriate:

(a) Immediate delivery of the fetus
(b) Intravenous quinine
(c) Intravenous quinine and intravenous chloroquine in combination
(d) Intravenous hydrocortisone
(e) The patient should be tested for G6PD deficiency before starting the quinine

26 (a) **False** – A broad spectrum pencillin
    (b) **False** – Should not be given to children under 12 years
    (c) **True**
    (d) **False** – Animal data suggest it causes arthropathy in growing joints
    (e) **False** – Inappropriate

27 (a) **True**
    (b) **True** – Chloramphenolol is also effective
    (c) **True** – Cefotaxime is also effective
    (d) **True**
    (e) **True** – Mebendazole is also effective in hookworm and roundworm
                  infections

28 (a) **False**   The aminoglycosides are effective in some Gram-positive and
    (b) **False**   many Gram-negative infections. They are not absorbed from
    (c) **True**   the gut, are principally eliminated in the urine and have a low
    (d) **True**   therapeutic ratio. Plasma drug concentrations should be
    (e) **False**   monitored.

29 (a) **True** – May be reduced by ondansetron or high dose metoclopramide
    (b) **False** – Occasionally causes gynecomastia
    (c) **True** – Treated with oral vancomycin or metronidazole
    (d) **False** – Used to treat AIDS-related Kaposi's sarcoma
    (e) **True** – Associated with cumulative dose when standard treatment
                  regimens are used

30 (a) **True**   Ethambutol and/or streptomycin are included if resistance is
    (b) **True**   predicted.
    (c) **True**
    (d) **False**
    (e) **False**

31 (a) **False**   Cerebral malaria has a particularly high morbidity/mortality in
    (b) **True**   pregnancy. Quinine is life-saving and must be initiated as
    (c) **False**   soon as possible.
    (d) **False**
    (e) **False**

32 The following are likely to be useful in reducing the plasma calcium concentration in a patient with severe hypercalcemia associated with myeloma:

(a) Intravenous saline
(b) Prednisolone
(c) Thiazide diuretics
(d) Tamoxifen
(e) Disodium etidronate

33 The following may be effective in the management of oral candidiasis:

(a) Nystatin
(b) Doxycycline
(c) Amphotericin
(d) Fluconazole
(e) Idoxuridine

34 Human insulin:

(a) Is usually produced from highly purified human pancreas
(b) Inhibits the subjective awareness of hypoglycemia
(c) Should not be given intravenously
(d) Is considerably more expensive than porcine insulin
(e) Should not be given concurrently with captopril

35 Allopurinol:

(a) Increases urinary elimination of uric acid
(b) Inhibits leukocyte migration
(c) Inhibits xanthine oxidase
(d) Reduces the plasma uric acid
(e) Should not be prescribed concurrently with a non-steroidal anti-inflammatory drug (NSAID)

36 The following drugs should be avoided in severe renal impairment:

(a) Prednisolone
(b) Oxytetracycline
(c) Metolazone
(d) Metformin
(e) Fybogel

37 Terfenadine:

(a) Is an H_1-receptor antagonist
(b) Should be avoided in significant hepatic impairment
(c) Metabolism is inhibited by ketoconazole
(d) Is associated with prolonged QT interval and torsade de pointes
(e) Is associated with hirsutism

32 **(a) True**   Severe hypercalcemia is a medical emergency. Initial and
    (b) True   immediate rehydration is essential.
    (c) False
    (d) False
    (e) True

33 **(a) True**   Broad-spectrum antibiotics, diabetes, inhaled steroids and
    (b) False   immunosuppression are predisposing factors in the develop-
    (c) True   ment of oral candidiasis.
    (d) True
    (e) False

34 **(a) False**   Human insulin can now be produced by recombinant
    (b) False   technology and is routinely used in newly diagnosed insulin-
    (c) False   dependent diabetics.
    (d) False
    (e) False

35 **(a) False**   Allopurinol is used prophylactically in the management of gout.
    (b) False   When allopurinol is started it may precipitate an acute attack,
    (c) True   hence it should be prescribed with an NSAID initially.
    (d) True
    (e) False

36 **(a) False**
    (b) True   – Antianabolic effect, increases urea, impairs renal function
    (c) False
    (d) True   – Increased risk of lactic acidosis
    (e) True   – Contains 7 mmol potassium per sachet

37 **(a) True**   Terfenadine is an over the counter (OTC) H_1-receptor
    (b) True   antagonist commonly used in the management of hayfever
    (c) True   and other allergic conditions. It only very rarely causes
    (d) True   sedation (cf. chlorpheniramine) but high plasma concentra-
    (e) False   tions prolong the QT interval.

38 A 16-year-old girl develops acute angioedema with stridor following an injection of intravenous ampicillin in the casualty department. The following are indicated:

   (a) Immediate intramuscular adrenaline
   (b) Intravenous serum C1 esterase inhibitor
   (c) Intravenous metoclopramide
   (d) Inhaled antihistamine
   (e) In addition to ampicillin, erythromycin should be avoided in the future

39 The following poisons have been paired with their appropriate antidotes:

   (a) Lead – penicillamine
   (b) Diamorphine – naloxone
   (c) DIazepam – flumazenil
   (d) Cyanide – dicobalt edetate
   (e) Propranolol – isoprenaline

40 A 20-year-old girl is admitted to the casualty department unconscious. There is reliable circumstantial evidence that she ingested 50 of her grandmother's amitriptyline tablets and 50 quinine tablets within the last hour. On admission, in addition to a grade IV coma, she has dilated pupils and brisk reflexes. Her blood pressure is 100/60, pulse 100 bpm. She is not cyanosed. Minute volumes and blood gases are acceptable. The ECG shows a wide QRS with prolonged QTc. The following are appropriate:

   (a) ECG monitoring
   (b) Stomach washout following placement of a cuffed endotracheal tube
   (c) Intravenous disopyramide
   (d) Forced acid diuresis
   (e) Stellate ganglion block to prevent blindness

41 A 14-year-old girl is seen in the A & E department. She is complaining of tinnitus and is hyperventilating and admits to having ingested a variety of at least 50 tablets from her parents' medicine cupboard, approximately 7 hours ago. The following statements are true:

   (a) Blood should be taken for salicylate concentration
   (b) Blood should be taken for paracetamol concentration
   (c) Blood should be taken for tricyclic antidepressant levels
   (d) Blood should be taken for benzodiazepine levels
   (e) An arterial sample should be taken for blood gas estimation

42 The management of a thyrotoxic crisis ("thyroid storm") usually requires treatment with:

   (a) Intravenous fluids
   (b) Propranolol
   (c) Hydrocortisone
   (d) Radioiodine (Iodine - 131)
   (e) Propylthiouracil

38 **(a) True**   In addition to intramuscular adrenaline, oxygen, intravenous
     (b) False   corticosteroids, intravenous fluids and intravenous
     (c) False   antihistamine are usually administered.
     (d) False
     (e) False

39 **(a) True**   – Sodium calcium edetate and dimercaprol (BAL) are also used.
                BAL is an effective antidote for most heavy metals. Desferri-
                oxamine is used in iron overdose
     (b) True
     (c) True
     (d) True   – Sodium nitrite followed by sodium thiosulfate are also used
     (e) True   – Intravenous atropine and glucagon are also effective

40 **(a) True**   Tricyclic antidepressants have a high mortality in overdose.
     (b) True   In addition to cardiac arrhythmias, convulsions are a recog-
     (c) False   nized potentially fatal complication.
     (d) False
     (e) False

41 **(a) True**   Patients who have taken a significant salicylate overdose
     (b) True   commonly present hyperventilating and complaining of
     (c) False   tinnitus. If there is a possibility of paracetamol overdose, its
     (d) False   plasma concentration should be measured as effective anti-
     (e) True   dotes are available.

42 **(a) True**   Thyrotoxic crisis requires emergency treatment. Carbimazole
     (b) True   or propylthiouracil may be administered by nasogastric tube if
     (c) True   the oral route is impractical. Propylthiouracil may be preferred
     (d) False   in "thyroid storm" because of its additional peripheral action
     (e) True   blocking conversion of T4 to T3. The hydrocortisone and
                propranolol are usually given by intravenous injection.

43 The following drugs commonly cause constipation:

    (a) Verapamil
    (b) Dihydrocodeine
    (c) Erythromycin
    (d) Misoprostol
    (e) Antacids containing aluminum

44 The combined oral contraceptive should not be prescribed if:

    (a) There is a history of severe or focal migraine
    (b) The girl is aged 16 and her parents have not consented
    (c) There is a history of deep vein thrombosis
    (d) Major elective surgery is planned within 4 weeks
    (e) There is a history of porphyria

45 Hormone replacement therapy is contraindicated if there is a history of:

    (a) Depression
    (b) Breast cancer
    (c) Deep vein thrombosis 20 years previously
    (d) Chronic obstructive bronchitis
    (e) Eczema

46 The following drugs are nephrotoxic:

    (a) Fluticasone
    (b) Cetirizine
    (c) Amikacin
    (d) Amphotericin B
    (e) Cyclosporin

47 The following drugs may precipitate bronchospasm:

    (a) Ibuprofen
    (b) Codeine phosphate
    (c) Labetalol
    (d) Aspirin
    (e) Adenosine

48 Non-steroidal anti-inflammatory drugs:

    (a) Reduce the effectiveness of loop diuretics
    (b) Reduce glomerular filtration in patients with glomerulonephritis
    (c) Impair the renal excretion of lithium
    (d) Are recognized causes of acute interstitial nephritis
    (e) Significantly increase urinary excretion of PGE_2

49 The following drugs are correctly paired with a recognized unwanted effect:

    (a) Vincristine and peripheral neuropathy
    (b) Nifedipine and peripheral edema
    (c) Cotrimoxazole and vitamin B_{12} deficiency
    (d) Metoclopramide and oculogyric crisis
    (e) Olsalazine and alopecia

43　(a) True
　　(b) True
　　(c) False
　　(d) False
　　(e) True

44　(a) True　　　The combined oral contraceptive should also be avoided
　　(b) False　　if there is undiagnosed vaginal bleeding, genital
　　(c) True　　　carcinoma, liver disease, valvular heart disease or a
　　(d) True　　　history of arterial embolism.
　　(e) True

45　(a) False　　In addition to preventing menopausal vasomotor
　　(b) True　　　symptoms and menopausal vaginitis if small doses of
　　(c) False　　estrogen are started in the perimenopausal period the
　　(d) False　　incidence of osteoporosis, stroke and myocardial
　　(e) False　　infarction are reduced. Unless the patient has had a hysterec-
　　　　　　　　tomy, a cyclic progestogen must be used to prevent the
　　　　　　　　increased risk of endometrial cancer.

46　(a) False – An inhaled/nasal corticosteroid
　　(b) False – An H_1-blocker
　　(c) True　 – Monitoring of aminoglycoside concentrations is mandatory in
　　　　　　　　renal impairment. Netilmicin may be the least nephrotoxic
　　　　　　　　aminoglycoside
　　(d) True　 – An antifungal agent often required in renal disease due to
　　　　　　　　immunosuppression
　　(e) True　 – An immunosuppressant used in the management of some
　　　　　　　　autoimmune diseases and transplantation

47　(a) True　 – All NSAIDs can precipitate bronchospasm in susceptible
　　　　　　　　asthmatics
　　(b) True　 – Opioids can precipitate bronchospasm
　　(c) True　 – A combined α- and β–blocker (β-blocking effects predominate)
　　(d) True
　　(e) True　 – Used in diagnosis/treatment of SVT

48　(a) True　　　NSAIDs should be avoided if possible in renal disease.
　　(b) True　　　The advantages of low dose aspirin in myocardial
　　(c) True　　　infarction and unstable angina generally outweigh any
　　(d) True　　　disadvantages.
　　(e) False

49　(a) True
　　(b) True　 – Largely unresponsive to diuretics
　　(c) False
　　(d) True　 – Treated with diazepam or an anticholinergic such as benztropine
　　(e) True

50 Drug induced hyperkalemia is caused by:

(a) Amiloride
(b) Spironolactone
(c) Enalapril
(d) Prednisolone
(e) Salbutamol

51 Ciprofloxacin:

(a) Has a large volume of distribution and penetrates tissues well
(b) Is effective in Gram-negative infection
(c) Inhibits cytochrome P_{450}
(d) Is concentrated in the urine
(e) Is useful for eradicating nasal carriage of *Meningococcus* in adults

52 Patients with G6PD deficiency may experience hemolysis from:

(a) Co-trimoxazole
(b) Succinylcholine
(c) Ciprofloxacin
(d) Halothane anesthesia
(e) Isoniazid

53 The following drugs cause pupil constriction (miosis):

(a) Dextropropoxyphene
(b) Neostigmine
(c) Amitriptyline
(d) Salbutamol
(e) Pilocarpine eye drops

54 Adverse effects associated with zidovudine (AZT) include:

(a) Neutrophilia
(b) Nausea and vomiting
(c) Myalgia
(d) Anemia
(e) Nephrotic syndrome

55 The following drugs cause hypertension:

(a) Corticosteroids
(b) Cyclosporin
(c) The oral contraceptive
(d) Imipramine
(e) Erythropoietin

56 The following drugs are associated with a facial "butterfly" rash:

(a) Nifedipine
(b) Phenytoin
(c) Captopril
(d) Isoniazid
(e) Prednisolone

50 (a) **True**
    (b) **True**
    (c) **True**
    (d) **False**
    (e) **False**

Drug-induced hyperkalemia is particularly dangerous if there is impaired renal function. The emergency treatment includes intravenous calcium chloride, intravenous glucose and insulin, sodium bicarbonate. To increase the elimination of potassium, calcium resonium and/or hemofiltration/hemodialysis are effective.

51 (a) **True**
    (b) **True**
    (c) **True**
    (d) **True**
    (e) **True**

Ciprofloxacin is a 4-fluoroquinolone which has broad-spectrum activity. It is particularly effective against Gram-negative bacteria but has only moderate activity against Gram-positive bacteria such as *Strep. pneumoniae* and *Strep. faecalis.*.It is well absorbed from the gut.

52 (a) **True**
    (b) **False**
    (c) **True**
    (d) **False**
    (e) **False**

Other drugs which induce hemolysis in most G6PD-deficient patients include dapsone, nitrofurantoin and primaquine.

53 (a) **True**
    (b) **True**
    (c) **False**
    (d) **False**
    (e) **True**

Pupil constriction is a sign of opioid overdose. Cholino-mimetics also cause miosis as does pontine hemorrhage. If there is asymmetry an intracerebral space occupying lesion (e.g. hematoma) or local lesion should be considered.

54 (a) **False**
    (b) **True**
    (c) **True**
    (d) **True**
    (e) **False**

AZT does not cure AIDS but may delay its progression. It is toxic.

55 (a) **True**
    (b) **True**
    (c) **True**
    (d) **False**
    (e) **True**

56 (a) **False**
    (b) **True**
    (c) **False**
    (d) **True**
    (e) **False**

Drug-induced SLE is usually reversible on withdrawing the causative drug.

57 The following drugs exert their therapeutic action by inhibition of the named enzyme:

   (a) Vigabatrin – GABA transaminase
   (b) Selegeline – dopa decarboxylase
   (c) Moclobemide – monoamine oxidase A
   (d) Acyclovir – RNA transcriptase
   (e) Enalapril – angiotension-converting enzyme

58 The following drugs may cause hypercalcemia:

   (a) Bendrofluazide
   (b) Frusemide
   (c) Calcitriol
   (d) Calcipotriol
   (e) Calcitonin

59 The following are recognized causes of neutropenia:

   (a) Prednisolone
   (b) Penicillamine
   (c) Mianserin
   (d) Clozapine
   (e) Cyclophosphamide

60 A 60-year-old man with a history of gout, diabetes and mild asthma (not requiring regular medication) is diagnosed as having essential hypertension. Which of the following drugs might be suitable?

   (a) Thiazide diuretic
   (b) Atenolol
   (c) Nifedipine
   (d) Captopril
   (e) Doxazosin

57 **(a) True**
    (b) False – Inhibits MAO-B
    (c) True
    (d) False – The triphosphate of acyclovir inhibits viral DNA synthesis
    (e) True

58 **(a) True**
    (b) False
    (c) True – A vitamin D derivative, 1,25-dihydroxycholecalciferol
    (d) True – A vitamin D derivative used topically in psoriasis
    (e) False

59 **(a) False**   Early appropriate drug withdrawal reduces the morbidity/
    (b) True   mortality. Granulocyte colony-stimulating factor (G-CSF) is
    (c) True   sometimes effective in the management of drug-induced
    (d) True   myelosuppression.
    (e) True

60 **(a) False** – Increases plasma urate and impaires glucose tolerance
    (b) False – Contraindicated in asthma (also masks subjective symptoms of
                    hypoglycemia)
    (c) True
    (d) True
    (e) True